GET MOVING!
LIVE BETTER, LIVE LONGER

GET MOVING!
LIVE BETTER, LIVE LONGER

Combat disease
with this medically
proven exercise guide

RUTH K. ANDERSON MD, MS

To order additional copies of this book, contact:
Xlibris Corporation
1-888-795-4274
www.Xlibris.com
Orders@Xlibris.com
66737

CONTENTS

ACKNOWLEDGMENTS

I realized two years ago that my diverse, often-disconnected background in wellness and disease really did have a purpose. The purpose is this book. I have been working toward its production for the past 30 years. No wonder, when I finally sat down to write it, the book wrote itself.

There are too many names to list, but I wish to thank all those who have affected its development along the way. Special thanks to Dr. Karl Stoedefalke who saw my potential in its rawest form 25 years ago and took a chance. He was the first to believe in me but not the last, and I thank you all. I also want to thank Jim Pawelczyk; he taught me that if you reach for the stars, you will grab one. Laura Kirkham was the initial push to get this book of the ground. And she is skilled at the art of 'push'. The list ends with all my patients—they were the ultimate inspiration for this book and the driving force to get it into print.

I must digress to share a little story. My two teenagers walked into the house one Saturday afternoon to find me, my laptop, and gazillion papers sprawled all over the dining room table. "Whatcha doin'?" they asked, laughing and wondering what the crazy lady was up to now. "Oh, I decided to write a book," I said like it was the most natural thing to do on a Saturday afternoon. They smiled their teenager smiles—not surprised, not even fazed—and went on their way. Without a complaint, they picked up all the slack at home and have been supportive every step of the way. All my love and thanks for covering any and all household chores and loving me even when I was a less-than-perfect mom. I am so blessed to share my life with Kate and Brad, two of the most intelligent, compassionate, independent people I have ever met. I will always be there to help you realize your dreams the way you have helped me realize mine.

A woman is nowhere without her friends, and I am nowhere without mine. Special thanks to David Auerbach who was at no loss for inspiration, even when I was. He is the unsung hero of this book and one of my most special friends. His production expertise made this book a reality. Gerri Reynolds has been my everlasting rock and salvation. Her wisdom and love guide me and strengthen me. I also want to thank my family for *always* being there. Always.

The photos were taken by Scott Avra of Avra Photography in Palm Desert, CA. His professionalism and dedication to his craft made for wonderful and very productive photo sessions. Couldn't have done it without him.

And lastly, I must thank one of the best physical therapists and one of the most amazing women I have ever worked with. Shelly Cooper donated her time, expertise, and even the use of her facility to make this book and my dream possible. She is in the photos at the end of each chapter along with Rick Raburn and Casey Casper. They are all stunning; I'm sure you'll agree.

INTRODUCTION

The odds are that you picked up this book because your doctor just told you that you're sick. Maybe you have just been diagnosed with hypertension, or you have elevated blood sugar—the first signs of diabetes. And he told you that you have 2 months to lose weight and start exercising, or you'll be on medication for the rest of your life. And then he wished you good luck, said good-bye and that he would see you in 3 months. Or maybe your dad just had a heart attack and you're afraid you'll end up the same way. You know what you need to do, but how do you start? Where do you turn?

Your doctor has diagnosed the problem and can provide pills to control your symptoms, but the power to improve your health rests solely with you. With an appropriately directed exercise program, you can take charge of your health. You can drop your blood pressure, treat your diabetes, strengthen your osteoporotic bones, and even control the pain of arthritis. You can actually fight your disease with the right exercise program, a program targeted to fight your specific medical problems. And in some instances, you can cure it. That is far more than modern medicine has to offer. You will see that you are more powerful than any pill your doctor can give you. I know; I'm one of the doctors that prescribe those pills. But I also know that your lifestyle choices, what you eat, and how you exercise are the best ways to treat and potentially cure your disease.

Modern medicine offers medications to treat the symptoms of disease but doesn't yet have the tools to cure disease. For example, we can control elevated blood sugar in diabetes, but unless you lose weight and exercise, you'll be taking those pills for the rest of your life. Exercise not only makes you look good and feel better, but it can also actually help you fight your disease. This book will teach you how to use exercise to fight your specific battles, to improve your health, and to significantly improve the quality of your life.

One very important example is the antihypertensive effect of exercise. Daily exercise can be as effective as any beta-blocker or calcium channel blocker in dropping your blood pressure. Think of it. It is actually possible to stop your medications with the right exercise program. Please don't stop taking your pills without your doctor's supervision, but as your blood pressure falls lower and lower with each office visit, your physician will be the first one to want to cut back on your medication. Less medication means fewer medication side effects (exercise is the only "medicine" without any) and lesser money out of your hard-earned paycheck as your monthly medical expenses drop. There is nothing but good news here.

So how do you fill the gap between your doctor's *strong* recommendation to exercise and finding someone to teach you the right way to do it? There are several places to turn. You could try the trainer at the gym, a physical therapist, or hope that you can catch enough time with your doctor to at least get an idea of where to start. But each specialist has his or her own focus, and none quite mesh with what you need. Trainers at the gym focus solely on how to train healthy young people. They are excellent at teaching healthy young adults how to exercise. But what if you're not 20? What if you're over 40 and recently diagnosed with sciatica, osteoporosis, or heart disease? Where do you turn? Your trainer clearly understands the mechanics of exercise, but he doesn't know how to use exercise to treat your specific disease. Nor does he have the exercise physiology background to help you exercise safely when you have arthritis, heart disease, or osteoporosis. Physical therapists are another option, but their expertise is specifically focused on helping you heal from an injury or surgery. So if you have an arthritic knee or have just had shoulder surgery, then they are the best step. But like the trainers at the gym, they do not have expertise in medical illnesses. On the other hand, your doctor is definitely the best person to direct the treatment of your disease, but his focus is on controlling your symptoms with medications, not on the ways exercise or diet can be used as a preventative medicine. And the way health care is changing (shrinking) in this country, there will be less time, not more, to focus on wellness—you must take charge of your own health, fitness, and nutrition. With this book in hand, you can focus on your health and effectively learn ways to use your time at the gym to make a significant impact on the quality of your life. Let your doctor focus on your disease, while you focus on your health and happiness.

One final reason and the most important in this economic climate is that maintaining your health and fitness is a monetary decision. There is less money than ever available for health care. So the sicker you choose to be, the more of your hard-earned dollars are going to pills and doctor visits. Poor choice. Fixable choice. And your choice starts here.

This book is the link, the link between what your doctors tells you to do and how to put it into action—safely and effectively. After reading the section on your specific disease(s), you will be able to go to the gym and exercise safely to achieve the gains you desire. You will also know that the time you spend exercising is a very efficient use of your time. This book provides a safe, medically based guide to start you on your way to health. This book is designed to be your first steps. My goal is to bridge the gap between your doctors telling you to exercise and the blank look on your face as you wonder what you're supposed to do to follow their advice.

I am writing this book because I believe that I can help you. I am an MD, board certified in both anesthesiology and pain management; I have a master's degree in exercise physiology, and I have a chronic low back pain. I have seen the medical profession from both sides (as a doctor and as a patient) and understand your frustration. I offer no hypes, no gimmicks, and have invented nothing new. The research in exercise physiology has been accumulating for over 50 years. All I am doing is taking my medical expertise and combining it with my 25 years' experience in health and wellness and my master's degree in exercise physiology to give you an easy-to-understand way to optimize your health.

What I have to offer is a scientifically based program that will work. It will work if you make the commitment one baby step at a time. No miracle results, no million dollars at the end of the rainbow, just a tried-and-true program that I've put into a form that you can incorporate into your life. What I do promise is that if you commit, then you will transform your life.

So taking one step at a time, let's get started.

NUTRITION BASICS TO
GET YOU STARTED

No wellness program is complete without some discussion of nutrition. You cannot optimize your health and treat your disease(s) without addressing both what you do and what you eat. Weight loss is of paramount importance to treat diabetes, hypertension, heart disease, arthritis, and even low back pain; and it's unlikely you can do it with exercise alone. In fact, for weight loss, how much you eat and what you eat are the most important factors for losing fat weight. Notice I put *how much you eat* first in that sentence—the quantity you eat should be foremost in your mind. Think about it. How many overweight people do you see at the gym? If exercise alone was enough, then we would all be lean and stay that way. But instead, month after month, we are running on the treadmill, and our spare tire never shrinks—yikes, it's actually getting bigger. That's because after 30 minutes of exercise (and my hat's off to all of you for sticking with it), you feel you have earned that 500-calorie muffin from Starbucks. The problem is, you only burned 250 calories. (I know, the calorie counters on the fancy exercise machine said you burned 600 calories, but they lie. Seriously, they do.) So your muffin put you 250 calories in fat debt; now add to that your daily mocha java latte smoothie and your 1,200-calorie diet is blown before you even get to work. We live in the land of plenty, and because of that, we have lost all sense of what real portions are. Exercise is critical for health; portion control is critical for fat loss and maintaining your optimal weight. Our life of convenience (translate that to high calorie, high fat, and high volume) is killing us. Think about this fact the next time you're at the drive-through window: you need to run

4 hours to burn off the calories in a single Big Mac. How much time do you realistically have in a day to exercise? Four hours? How much do you really like to run? I stopped eating Big Macs after I read that—I hate to run. Diet and exercise must go hand in hand for you to quickly reach your health goals. Now, while I am trying hard to drive home the point that you can't use exercise alone to shrink your waistline, don't let me discount the value of physical activity in helping you reach your goals. The right exercise program will increase your muscle mass so that it is easier to burn calories and keep them off for good. It's the combination of portion control and exercise that will succeed.

Over the years, exercise and diet fads have come and gone, and then they come back again. The Atkins diet failed in the 1970s and again in the 1990s (if it was truly successful, then we'd all have been thin by 1980, right?), and I'm sure it will be recycled several more times before we finally put it and all the other fads to rest. We grab on to these gimmicks trying to find answers, but the truth gets lost in the media and advertising hype. So put away the Ab Blaster, your cabbage soup diet, and the Hydroxycut pills because you know we're no thinner or healthier now than we were in the 1970s. Actually, we're in much worse shape. We're sicker, more obese, and more sedentary than ever. There are no magic pills in the world of fitness, nutrition, or medicine. If the promises of quick painless weight loss or rapid muscle growth sound too good to be true, then you can bet they are.

The amazing thing about the nutrition principles to follow is that they apply to all the diseases discussed in this book—the diseases of modern society. And that's not hype—it's hard science. And it is so simple, really. The more we learn about disease, the more we realize that there is a common denominator to most diseases known today. This common denominator is inflammation and it presents in many ways; in heart disease, the result is a heart attack, and in chronic pain, the end result is unrelenting suffering. But the instigator is the same. We are learning that many diseases originate from inflammatory processes at the cellular level. We now understand that heart disease is caused by more than just the fat you eat. It appears that a diet that promotes inflammation in our bodies can lead to all types of illness from heart disease to certain cancers to chronic pain. And the typical American diet is just that—the diet that promotes inflammation in our bodies. This inflammation destroys the integrity of each cell and causes disease. The typical American diet is pro-inflammation. It is the wrong way to eat. It is a diet high in the bad fats called saturated or trans fat and low in the good fats like olive and canola oil. Our diet is dependent on processed foods and lacking in foods found in their natural state. You will hear more and more about an anti-inflammatory diet as the way to combat disease in the years to come. This is not a diet per se. Most of the tenets of an anti-inflammatory diet fit perfectly with the long-standing recommendations of eating a low-fat high-fiber diet. So it's not really new. It is what wellness experts have advocated since the 1970s. But as we learn more about wellness, we are fine-tuning the old standby. Diets advocated by the American Heart Association and the American Cancer Society are good examples of this way of eating. There is no hype and no gimmicks. And no one is getting rich off it, so you won't see it widely advertised. But it is sound science that has stood the rigors of years of success. The guidelines below are based on this science. They give you a way to live your life to increase your energy level, maintain or lose weight, and optimize your health.

So despite all the health gimmicks, there are nutrition and exercise basics that have never changed and never been disproved. They are the golden rules of health and wellness and are the keys for you to live a long and happy life—a life full of vitality.

Golden Rule 1. A diet based on fruits, vegetables, and whole grains will sustain the health you were born with.

You were born healthy. Don't muck it up with a bunch of fast foods and processed foods. Eating real foods will help you fight a whole slew of diseases from heart disease to colon cancer to diabetes. There is no other diet that has been shown to fight disease. Over the past 30-plus years, more and more research has accumulated to support the health benefits of this diet. This healthy way to eat is much less flashy than the diet fads listed on the NY Times best seller list, but these sound eating habits have withstood the rigors of science and time. It is simple: Do your grocery shopping around the perimeter of the grocery store. Avoid the isles in the middle of the store packed full of processed food and badness. Fill your shopping cart with foods in their natural state, like what you get in the produce section, the meat counter, and the dairy section of the grocery store (but pick the lower-fat dairy and meat selections, please). Base your meals around what you purchase at the local farmers' market. But remember frozen and canned vegetables are as healthy as fresh and just as good for you.

Carbohydrates are not bad and have never been bad; the fiber in whole grain bread and cereals is important for GI health and cancer prevention. Atkins did us no favors. Eat whole grains and minimize or avoid refined grains like white bread and packaged crackers and snack foods (again, avoiding the processed foods). Instead, choose brown rice and whole grains (read the ingredient list, please, packaging is deceptive), which offer tons of fiber and trace elements required for good health. Pick products that offer at least four grams of fiber per serving. The highly processed carbohydrates like donuts and cake are the ones to avoid, but not because it's a carbohydrate, but because they are filled with fat and sugar. I am diametrically opposed to processed foods, but I have found a few that may actually help your weight control and keep you from being a slave to the kitchen. I am a big fan of Fiber One bars. They keep my daily caloric intake low and still fill me up. They are the only processed foods I eat.

Golden Rule 2. Keep your meals full of color.

Reds, greens, yellows. You see, the more colorful your diet, the greater variety of nutrients you are getting. A multivitamin can help in a crunch, but they don't contain everything your body needs to function and fight disease. The truth is, we still know so little about the human body, about disease, and about health. What we know is that over the years, we have discovered so many trace elements that are critical for optimal health that the only way to be assured you are getting all the elements we haven't discovered yet (because believe me, there is a book full just waiting to be found) is to eat a diet that is rich in color and variety. No pill will give you what you need, no matter what the bottle promises. But you'll find it in nature. So eat a variety of foods to get the necessary vitamins, minerals, and antioxidants that you can't get from any other. Regardless of the outrageous claims of the health food stores, only Mother Nature can guarantee complete health.

Golden Rule 3 (and my favorite). Everything in moderation including moderation.

A very wise man once said that, and it has stuck with me since graduate school. I eat well and make healthy choices because they make me feel good. And I eat healthy the majority of the time. But when I want to splurge, I do. And I don't think twice about a piece of chocolate cake (OK, I think twice, but that's it). I don't need to obsess about the number of calories I ate that day because I choose to live healthy and make smart choices the other 85%–90% of the time. You must find your balance. Moderation is great for health and life, but if you don't treasure your guilty pleasures, then life is only half as good. And I can guarantee that if you deprive yourself of foods that give you joy, then you will fall off the health bandwagon before its wheels even get rolling. How many have failed the cabbage soup diet? the grapefruit diet? the Atkins diet? Need I continue? With that said, you need to read Golden Rule 4. I hope you find a way to make it true for you.

Golden Rule 4. Start to find ways to make your healthy choices self-fulfilling.

I eat fruits and vegetables because they make me feel good. Your healthy choices of food will make you feel strong and light and energized like they do for me. In my 20s, I taught myself to rethink my approach to food. I gave up Big Macs and Cap'n Crunch's Crunch Berries (my childhood favorites) but not because I was depriving myself or decided to become a martyr in the name of health. I started to look at them differently. Although eating them was fun, they made me tired and bloated and fat, and I would continually tell myself that's how they made me feel. And pretty soon, I lost my craving for them, and instead, I started to make food choices that made me feel strong and invigorated. And I kept telling myself my healthy choices made me feel good until they really did. I don't eat healthy as a sacrifice. Instead, I trained myself and talked to myself so that I started to prefer healthy foods and saw eating healthy foods as a reward. And the reward is health, strength, and a lean body that can meet all the daily challenges I face. And that lean body looks darn good—so will yours. With every healthy choice I made, I felt more and more in control of my life, my health, and my future. If you spend your days focusing on what you gave up instead of on the positive and rewarding choices you make, then you will never make the transition to a healthy life. You will never regain the health and wellness you were born with, and you definitely will never keep it.

So you need to start with modest adjustments to your food choices. Baby steps most often lead to permanent change. And you've heard them all before, so I won't belabor the point. But a simple example is to change from whole milk to 2% to eventually skim milk. You have all the calcium, protein, and vitamins without any of the fat. Calcium actually helps with weight loss if you choose the low-fat varieties. And calcium obtained in dairy products is much more effective at treating and preventing osteoporosis than calcium in pill form because vitamin D is coupled with it. But the best source of vitamin D is the sun. Fifteen minutes every day will provide the most bioavailable form of this nutrient. So sunshine in moderation is necessary for health. In excess, it can cause cancer, but moderation is the key.

But remember, the important adjustment you can make to your eating habits is portion control. This is by far the most important change you can make. For example, over the past 20 years, the size of the plate restaurants serve dinner on has increased from 9 inches to 13 inches, and they are packed with more food than ever. We're eating 25%–30% more food at each sitting and haven't even realized it. How many times have you heard a friend talk about a great restaurant not because of the quality of food it serves but because you get so much food for your money? You have got to rethink your definition of quality. And remember, every extra calorie you eat that you don't burn off turns to fat. If you don't burn it off, then it will be stored away as fat for a rainy day. The problem is that we no longer have rainy days. So the fat just keeps accumulating. Quantity is killing us. We are overeating ourselves to death.

If you think about it, the basics of nutrition are very simple and easy to remember. No fads, no gimmicks, no pot of gold. Just solid science and practical advice to get you on the right track. I refer you to the Harvard School of Public Health and their healthy eating pyramid. It provides an easy-to-follow guide to choosing a healthy diet: http://www.hsph. harvard.edu/nutritionsource/what-should-you-eat/.

Or you can visit the Mayo Clinic Web site: http://www.mayoclinic.com. Select the Healthy Lifestyle section (upper right option on the home page). This will direct you to a wealth of information on nutrition, fitness, and weight loss.

Both Web sites give you practical guidance with a sound scientific base. I strongly recommend both.

GENERAL EXERCISE PRINCIPLES

So you have been given the *very* strong suggestion by your doctor to lose weight and exercise, and you're ready to give it a try. You should be proud of yourself for taking the most important step. Here is where you start. And we will start together. This chapter gives you a brief understanding of exercise basics. This is the foundation you need to understand the following chapters that discuss how exercise is used to treat disease. After reading this, you should then turn to the chapter or chapters that correspond to your specific medical problems and get started. Feel free to refer back to this chapter for reinforcement as needed.

Before we talk about exercise, I want you to understand the importance of movement. It is equally important for you to increase the amount you move each day as it is to commit time to your official exercise sessions. I am modifying the phrase "use it or lose it" to become your new mantra. It's now "move it or lose it." And you must move it. And you must keep it moving, or you will lose your strength, vitality, and your ability to care for yourself as you grow older.

Moving is your best hedge against aging. Note I used the term *moving*, not *exercise*. All you need to do is move. I'm talking about simply increasing your activity level. Bit by bit. For example, park away from the mall entrance and walk the distance of the parking lot, take the stairs instead of the elevator, and dance to the radio while you brush your teeth. Just move. Increase the amount of time you move in a day, and you will dramatically impact your health and make a real dent in your weight loss program. Growing old is inevitable, but there is no reason you can't do it well and with joy. Unfortunately, as we grow older and get busier with the demands of life, we naturally get less active. When was the last time you climbed a tree? Or for that matter, when was the last time your kids climbed a tree? We're less and less active. It's a recipe for disaster. I have made myself a few rules to help fight this aging tendency in myself. And I want to share them with you. I keep simple tasks a challenge, and I stay strong. You can use mine or pick your own; the effect will be the same. For example, I will not sit in a chair to put on my shoes. I work on my balance every day as I stand on one leg to put on my shoes and socks. Balance and falls are a terrible problem in the elderly, primarily because they are weak and don't practice balance skills. Don't give in to the chair. Challenge your balance daily. Another one of my rules is that I never use my arms to help me get out of a chair—only my legs. This keeps my thigh muscles strong, burns a few more calories each day, and avoids knee pain. Every patient that sits in my office pushes themselves out of the chair with their arms. And they wonder why they have no leg strength, sore knees, and bad balance. Think about how you move through the day. You will be shocked at how you have reduced your activity over the years to make your life easier. But remember, easier translates into weaker muscles and more body fat and a real struggle to live independently as you grow old. Children know the secret. They move for maximal energy burn. They run, skip, or hop when expected to walk. They have the right idea. Next time you walk down the hall at home, do some lunges or gentle leg lifts instead of just trudging along. Or brush your teeth standing on one leg. I give you these suggestions so you'll realize that you can challenge yourself on a daily basis and, by doing these simple things, keep yourself strong, independent, and fit well into your 80s and 90s.

So now you are moving. Every day. That is definitely the place to start. But that is just the start. You need to incorporate effective exercise into your weekly schedule. There are several basic principles of exercise of which you should be aware. The most important principle is that your success hinges on finding ways to make this book work for you. Your *most* important job is to find what you enjoy. You should walk if it brings you joy. But if it doesn't and dancing does, then by all means dance. There are no temporary fixes; you need a permanent solution to maintain your health from now till you are in your 90s. So please find what makes you happy. Any of the *-ing* words work for aerobic exercise. Walking, running, biking, swimming are but a few examples.

The -ing words that don't apply are sitting and sleeping—obviously. So go find the -ing you love. And in the process, find your inner child and enjoy the trial and error of learning something new. In the chapters to come, I will take the -ing exercises that you enjoy and create an exercise program that is specifically targeted to your disease. So bear with me now. These principles may be a bit dry, but I feel strongly that a few basics will provide the groundwork for you to understand what you need to do and why you are doing it. Depending on what medical problems you have, I will create an exercise program for you using 4 different phases. These include your warm-up, aerobic exercise (the -ing words), weight training, and then cooldown. Depending on your medical problems, these phases take on a different importance. For example, arthritis patients should focus on weight training to build muscle to support their aching joints, whereas heart patients should do primarily aerobic exercise. Let's review the important considerations in each phase. The first is warm-up.

WARM-UP

The warm-up period is one of the most important parts of your exercise program because it helps your body prepare for the rigors of exercise and prevents injury. It increases blood flow to your working muscles, decreases muscle and joint stiffness, and limbers up tendons and ligaments in preparation for more strenuous work. It literally warms up your body (increasing your body temperature). And as your body warms up, your muscles, tendons, and ligaments warm up, which will decrease stiffness and help prevent injury. The proper warm-up also introduces your heart and cardiovascular system to the stress of exercise by gradually increasing blood flow to the heart, which will minimize exercise-induced cardiac problems. Think of your warm-up as the TLC you are giving your body so it can meet the demands of your exercise session yet to come.

Start with an easy walk and progress to a brisk pace with your arms swinging. This will gradually increase your body temperature and literally warm up your muscles and your joints. You want to get your blood flowing and your heart pumping. If you have any problem or painful areas, then this is a good time to give them a bit of tender loving care—make sure you do a few specific stretches for these trouble areas. I think the best warm-up is simply walking outside in the fresh air for 5–10 minutes at a progressively faster pace. By the time the 10 minutes is done, you should be breathing harder and feeling that your body is warm. Another way to warm up is to do one set of your weight training exercises using about half your usual weight and quickly run through a full-body workout. Anything that gets your blood flowing and your breathing heavy is a good warm-up.

AEROBIC EXERCISE

Aerobic exercise is the cornerstone of your exercise program designed to fight the diseases of modern society. It's been the exercise buzzword for 30-plus years, and there is a good reason. It works. It works for heart health, weight loss, cholesterol lowering, and stress reduction, just to name a few. It is still the cornerstone of exercise science because it works and it has stood the test of time. Think about it, what pill or supplement or diet fad has this kind of staying power and this amount of supporting research behind it? Nothing. Aerobic exercise—*cardio* as the lingo goes—is any of the *-ing* words. They include *walking, jogging, biking, rowing, hiking, dancing, stair climbing*, and even *skipping*. The only *-ing* words that don't count are *sitting* and *lying down*. They won't do a darn thing for your heart.

Aerobic exercise specifically trains the heart and cardiovascular system. Because your heart is a muscle just like any other muscle in your body, it gets bigger and stronger with stress. Aerobic exercise gives your heart the right kind of stress to make it bigger and stronger. A strong heart is a healthy heart. Aerobic exercise also strengthens all your other muscles and makes them more efficient. In addition, and this is really good news, with regular aerobic exercise, your body gets more efficient at using stored fat as the fuel for exercise. Fat burning is a goal for all of us. So making a commitment to a regular aerobic exercise program will go far in helping you achieve your weight loss goals. As your body gets strong and efficient, you will increase your fitness reserve. That means that you can carry out your daily activities much easier because you have a reserve to pull from. Sedentary individuals who are not very fit find that simple things, like carrying in the groceries or even walking into the grocery store, are exhausting because of their low reserve. As you get aerobically fit, you will have much more reserve to pull from, and groceries will be a breeze. Building your reserve, a reserve of strength and a reserve of heart health, is critical to help you stay healthy and independent as you grow old. If you have been sedentary, then it will take nothing more than just a simple walking program to see significant gains.

So you have found what you enjoy. The next questions are how hard, how long, and how often you should exercise. I believe that one of the biggest reasons people fail to stick with their exercise program is that they don't know how to optimize their time in the gym. And they realize this. They know they aren't using their time effectively, and so they stop going. Why waste 3–5 hours at the gym each week if you can't be sure that you're getting everything out of it than you should? I have customized each exercise program to fight your medical problems and optimize your health. You will know that your time in the gym is well spent, and that will keep you focused and motivated.

The first principle is intensity, or simply how hard you are exercising. The most accurate way to determine how hard you are exercising is to monitor your heart rate—you will see it referred to as your target heart rate range. However, it has limitations, so don't go out and buy a heart rate monitor. We can get a good estimation by monitoring three parameters: your breathing rate, whether you can talk during exercise, and your perception of how hard you're working. For example, light-intensity exercise is the neighborhood ladies out for their morning constitutional; they are chitchatting away and not even breaking a sweat. Generally, light-intensity exercise is a waste of your precious time. But there are a few specific groups of patients who can see significant health gains with even this lowest level of exercise. These are chronic pain patients who have been very sedentary secondary to their pain, patients with significant heart disease, and all of you exercise virgins. You see, the more out of shape you are, the quicker you will benefit from even the least amount of exertion. Not necessarily a good thing, but a reality. In each chapter, I will discuss an optimum intensity at which you should be exercising to achieve your specific goals.

Exercise physiologists quantify how hard you are working several ways. My favorite is your perception of how hard you are working, and we use a scale to express it. But you can also use a heart rate monitor and the table below. Let's talk a little more about the perceived exertion scale (the Borg scale, after its inventor). You can tell how hard you're working by monitoring your breathing rate and your overall sense of how hard you are exercising. To exercise at a light-to-moderate intensity, you should walk at a speed fast enough that you know you are exercising but not so fast that your are unable to easily have a conversation with yourself or your workout partner (a 5/10 on the perceived exertion scale). If a slow stroll is too easy, then increase your pace. Moderate exercise intensity (7/10) is when you are breathing hard but you can still talk but with difficulty. Here's your guide:

Perceived Exertion Scale

1/10	Sitting and watching TV
3/10	Exercising comfortably but breathing a bit hard
5/10	Exercising just above your comfort level, but you can still have a conversation easily
7/10	Sweating like a pig, but you can still talk
9/10	I won't last another 30 seconds, this has got to stop
10/10	Death must feel better than this

A second way to monitor your exercise intensity is to use a heart rate monitor. The table below gives the safe and appropriate heart rate range to exercise for your age. Besides only being an estimate of what is your intensity range, there are other reasons why monitoring your heart rate is less than ideal. Many heart and blood pressure medications blunt the heart rate response to exercise. You may be working at a 6–7/10 intensity level, but your heart rate won't approach the range listed below because of certain medications you are taking, such as beta-blockers. So I strongly recommend that you listen to your body and worry less about an actual heart rate number. In addition, the accuracy of your heart rate monitor can be affected by your movement, so it may or may not be accurate. Please use the table below as a rough guide.

Target Heart Rate Table

Age   *Target Heart Rate Range*

(50%–85% exercise intensity)

30 years	95–162 bpm
35 years	93–157 bpm
40 years	90–153 bpm
45 years	88–149 bpm
50 years	85–145 bpm

55 years	83–140 bpm
60 years	80–136 bpm
65 years	78–132 bpm
70 years	75–128 bpm

As your fitness level improves over the weeks and months to follow, you will need to increase how hard you are exercising to continue to see fitness and health gains. If you don't continue to challenge your body, then you will not continue to grow. So remember, complacency is your enemy. As you become more fit, you'll need to move faster to keep breathing heavy and stay within your target range. Consequently you will go further as your fitness level improves. This is the best indication that your heart and cardiovascular system are getting stronger. That is why I like the breathing method so much. Heavy breathing is your key. Dr. Ruth is all for heavy breathing. So again, your eventual exercise intensity goal is to be breathing hard, but not so hard that you can't carry on a conversation. Your long-term goal is to not fall into a rut of walking 30 minutes and a set distance without continually pushing to increase the distance you can go in that time. Each chapter will discuss the optimal exercise intensity to treat your disease and how to progress safely to optimize your health gains.

Anyone who is sedentary and beginning an exercise program for the first time should start at a very low intensity (40%–50% maximum or a perceived exertion of 4–5) and gradually increase your effort as tolerated. A regular exercise program safeguards against the risk of sudden death, but you need to build your safety net slowly so the safeguard doesn't become the trigger. With a regular exercise program, you have significantly decreased your chance of dying with any vigorous activity—be it shoveling snow or having wild sex. If you have a clean bill of health from your doctor regardless of your age *and* have been exercising on a regular basis, then I recommend an intensity level of 50%–70% of your maximum ability. This corresponds to a perceived exertion score of 5–7. As you get more fit over the next 6 months, you can increase the intensity of your exercise session so that the majority of the time you are in the "sweating like a pig" range (a 7 on the Borg scale).

The second principle is frequency, or how often you should exercise. You have all heard that you should exercise 3–4 days a week. You're right.

This is based on strong evidence that it requires at least 3 days a week of exercise to see changes in health and fitness. All the experts agree that your body needs days off to rest and recover, preferably spread out through the week rather than clumped together. If you exercise every day of the week, then you will defeat your purpose. You will increase your fatigue level, compromise your immune system, and tear down the muscles you are trying to build. Your body must have several days of rest to rebuild at a newer, stronger level. And your 2 days of rest should be scattered through the week and not back-to-back. However, I think the most important thing about frequency is the time you can realistically commit. Any commitment is better than none. One day a week is better than nothing. Really, it is. Our biggest problem in our society is that we have stopped moving. Just move. Remember that 2 minutes of deep knee bends while you are brushing your teeth is movement. And the more you move each day, the more your frequency of exercise will increase and the faster your waistline will decrease. A brisk walk after dinner counts, so do those teeth-brushing knee bends or dancing to the radio as you brush your hair.

The third principle is duration, how long you should exercise. After a 5-minute warm-up, you must exercise for at least 12 minutes at moderate intensity to see fitness gains. Then follow up your aerobic session with a 5-minute cooldown. That is the bare-bones basics. Twenty-two minutes 3 times a week to see fitness gains. Not bad. You could do better, but that's a great start. The fitness gains I'm talking about consist of strengthening your cardiovascular system and lungs and building more muscle mass. That's not a lot—just the bare minimum for health. A more desirable goal is 30–40 minutes 3–4 days a week. But I don't want you jumping off the couch today and running at 70% intensity for 30 minutes. You may be able to do it, but I can promise you, if you are new to exercise, then you won't be walking well for the next week. And then you'll quit. Start low and go slow. It is how I titrate my patient's medication, and it's how you should gently introduce your body to exercise. Your muscles will adapt fairly quickly to the demands of your new exercise program. And they will adapt much quicker than your ligaments, tendons, and joints. That's where the injuries usually occur. Gradually increase your exercise duration/intensity and frequency so that all body tissues have time to strengthen and adapt. It's too easy to overdo it and let an injury derail all your good intentions. Patience and gradual progress are much harder to accept, but are the way to go for lasting success. Go slow, go steady, and you will see the results you seek. A very wise man once said, "Infinite patience will yield immediate results." Your results will come, and the benefits will be beyond your wildest dreams—benefits that arise from your willingness to take control of your life and your health and, most importantly, from your belief that you are worth the effort.

Now, how are these parameters modified for people with different diseases? That we will cover in the chapters to come. Keep these 3 basic principles in mind when you exercise so you exercise safely and effectively to achieve your goals of health and happiness with maximum efficiency.

You will hear me talk about body posture and alignment throughout this book. Maybe it's because I'm a pain management specialist and know that 70% of you will suffer back pain in your life. Or maybe it's because I spent the first 22 years of my life as a dancer. Regardless, I know how important proper form is to prevent injury, heal your pain, and optimize each workout. While you are doing your aerobic exercise, stand tall with your stomach muscles firm to support your back. Try to keep your stomach muscles contracted the entire walk. Think of how you would tense your stomach if someone was going to punch you in the gut. When they come at you with that fist, you don't pull away but tighten your stomach to brace for the hit. Or you can try saying *sshhh*. Try it right now and say it loud so you really have to engage your core. This is another way to tighten your gut and engage the deep core muscles to protect your back. The more you *sshhh* yourself, the stronger these critical muscles become and the better you look. Playtex did us no favors by popularizing the girdle. To get the most out of your exercise session, you must be your own Playtex girdle. The girdle did nothing but take away our responsibility for a firm, strong core. Abdominal crunches don't build a strong core. They only strengthen the outermost abdominal muscle (the rectus abdominis) that gives you a nice six-pack. But crunches don't strengthen the deeper 3 sets of abdominal muscles that comprise your true core. The way to train them is to act like a boxer bracing for a punch in the gut or to just say *sshhh*.

Now you know everything you need to know about cardio. It's time to get to the weight room.

RESISTANCE TRAINING

The other important focus of your exercise program must be resistance training. And by that I mean weight lifting. Back in the 1970s and 1980s, we thought that aerobic training was the ticket to health and wellness. We have learned that to be healthy and grow old well, you must fight the inevitable loss of muscle mass that happens as we get more sedentary with age. It's not the growing-old part that causes muscle wasting; it is our lack of activity and exercise. What we know now is that decreased muscle mass is associated with poor function of your immune system, the onset of heart disease and diabetes, weaker bones, stiffer joints, and a slumped posture. Muscle only grows when you stress it. If you spend your days sitting on the couch and pushing yourself out of the chair with your arms, then you will experience a yearly loss of muscle mass that really accelerates after the age of 50. Since we no longer spend our days driving a plow in the fields or throwing bales of hay, you have got to find other means to work your muscles. Barbells are perfect. Each chapter of my book ends with resistance exercises for this very reason. You need to stay strong to be healthy and grow old the best way you can. Watching my mother age was a real inspiration to me, but not in the good sense. I remember coming home from college and watching the woman who used to bound up the stairs now struggle with each step. She had to put her hand on each knee to find the strength to lift her body up to the next step. And she was only in her 50s. She wasn't sick, but she had never exercised and now didn't have the strength in her thighs to even lift her own body weight. I decided right then that I would never be so weak that I couldn't carry in my own groceries, run up the stairs, or climb a ladder to change a light bulb. All these things you take for granted, but I see them lost every day in my elderly patients who are having trouble caring for themselves. The more we learn about health, the more we learn that maintaining your muscle mass (or finding it again if you lost it) is critical. Modern medicine is doing a great job at helping us live longer, but we don't yet have that pill to make those extra years wonderful. All my patients ask what happened to the golden years? They have the years, but they aren't that golden. You have the power to make them golden, but you have to start now. Not tomorrow.

As we age and become less active, we lose muscle at an alarming rate. This loss of muscle mass and fall in resting metabolic rate is not an inevitable result of aging. It is a result of our inactivity and our sedentary lifestyle. By weight training 3 days a week, you can reverse this loss. Studies have shown that people over the age of 70 can still get stronger with a weight training program—you are never too old to start.

Resistance training will increase your muscle mass, and with more muscle, you have a higher resting metabolic rate. That means you are burning more calories with everything that you do. The more muscle you have, the more calories your body is burning even when sitting and watching TV. Muscle is metabolically active tissue—it is burning calories 24 hours a day. Fat just sits there and puts an undue stress on your heart, on your back, and on your joints. Even more important, the stronger you are and the healthier you feel, the more active you will be each day just because you feel better. You'll walk just a little faster, hold your body up a little straighter, and all these subtle changes will make a big impact in your daily calorie burning. By burning those extra calories on a 24-7 basis, you will start to see those inches whittle away. But most important, as you get stronger, simply moving and living become much easier. So you move more and you live more. Every day as your joy with life increases, so does your calorie burning. Not a bad way to change your life for the better.

Another important benefit of weight training is its effect on blood sugar control. Diabetes is a significant risk factor for heart disease and accompanies high blood pressure at an alarming rate. With exercise (not just aerobic exercise), you can attack diabetes and coronary artery disease. Weight training leads to improved glucose control and also improves the ability of insulin to do its job. Your body needs insulin to drive blood sugar out of the blood and into each cell where it is used for fuel. It is high levels of sugar in your blood (not in your cells) that does all the damage we see with diabetes—blindness, kidney failure, and peripheral neuropathy to name a few. In type 2 diabetes, the problem is increased insulin resistance; in other words, your cells won't let insulin do its job. Exercise works in your favor and lowers your body's insulin resistance so the cells will let it in.

Now you know weight training is beneficial on many levels. It will improve your heart health, shrink your waistline, and even help control your blood sugar. And I didn't even mention its ability to treat depression, control anxiety, and combat chronic pain. And I could go on and on.

In addition, you will find that your aerobic exercise (whether you chose walking, biking, or swimming) will be much easier as you build muscle strength with weight training. Weight training will keep your bones strong, and it will improve your balance. It is the force of muscle pulling against bone that stimulates bone growth and fights osteoporosis. One in three Americans over the age of 65 fall every year. Resistance exercise cannot only improve your balance but will also decrease your risk of falling and strengthen your bones in case you do.

The importance of balance cannot be emphasized enough. Balance is a skill, a skill you will lose if you don't practice. So brush your teeth standing on one leg, and when that is easy, do it with your eye closed. To improve your balance, you need to do exercises specifically targeted to your balance problems. For example, if you are unsteady while walking, then exercises that require you balance on one leg will strengthen the muscles you need. I have included balance exercises at the end of the section on leg exercises. Please make sure you can do the exercises perfectly on two feet before you try them on one.

Generally, exercise physiologists recommend 2–3 weight training sessions per week. This will vary depending on your medical problems. I believe that a circuit approach is the way to get the most out of your exercise time. I do one exercise for each muscle group without resting. No need for chitchat between each exercise. Keep your body moving, and the muscles you last worked will rest as you use different muscles in the next exercise. This not only maximizes your use of time, but also gives your heart a little boost because you never let your heart rate slow down. If you are new to resistance work, then you can probably work your entire body (upper and lower) during each exercise session.

For generalized strengthening and toning, don't spend an entire exercise session on your biceps and triceps. This is counterproductive. If you want to lose your flabby arms, then lose the fat lying over them that is jiggling in the breeze. And that won't happen by doing 50 triceps curls or even 50,000. To lose the jiggle, you must drop your body fat. The best way to drop fat is to pick exercises that work several large muscle groups during each weight training session so you will burn more calories. In fact, you really don't have to spend any time on biceps and triceps since they will get strong when you do push-ups, pull-ups, and all the other exercises that train multiple large muscle groups.

I train my entire upper body or my lower body each time I'm at the gym. Also, I never rest between exercises, so my heart rate stays elevated, and I get a bit of aerobic work even when I'm weight lifting. I am in and out of the gym in 30–45 minutes and much stronger and well-defined than most others who spend 2 hours in a less productive workout. Think of the approach as a circuit. Move from one exercise to another without a break. I am working hard and breathing heavy throughout my exercise session. Dr. Ruth does like heavy breathing.

It is easy to fall into bad exercise habits, especially when it comes to weight lifting. The following is a list of common mistakes that waste time and can be dangerous if you are not in perfect health. I have probably seen every mistake in the book, but these are the most common and the ones you need to avoid:

1. Failing to monitor your progress

Use a training log to monitor your progress and help you achieve your goals. This is a very important step especially for beginners because we know that when you have goals, the chances of sticking with your exercise program is increased significantly. And this needs to be a life commitment.

2. Lifting weight that is too heavy

You must be able to control your weight through the entire exercise and have perfect form throughout the entire exercise. When you start to lose your form, it is time to end the set. Lifting a weight that is too heavy puts too much stress on your joints, tendons, and ligaments, but it also puts too much stress on your heart. This is dangerous when you have high blood pressure or heart disease. You'll know the weight is too heavy when you are straining and have stopped breathing or when you start to lose your form.

3. Doing the same routine every workout session

Muscles get accustomed to the same exercises, and the benefit from doing the same routine over and over diminishes over time. Muscles do get bigger and stronger when they are challenged with new exercises. In addition to trying new exercises, muscles also get stronger when you change the speed that you do the exercises and the order that you do your exercises. For example, for your upper body workout, start one day with chest, the next with back or shoulders. One week, lift weight to the count of 2; the next week, slow everything down to the count of 4 or 8.

4. Using incorrect form

I stress exercising with a partner so they can monitor your form. In addition, you should use the mirrors in the gym to check your body alignment (not to admire your biceps). Pay attention that your low back isn't rounded, your stomach is taut, your shoulders are back, and your low back has its normal curvature. Also, make sure you keep your body stable during each exercise (core engaged) and don't use your torso to help you move the weight. I'm sure you've all seen the guy at the gym that swings his whole body to do a bicep curl with a weight that is way too heavy for him. He is risking injury and not getting much benefit from the exercise since momentum is doing all the work. Now who's the dumbbell in that exercise?

5. Focusing on what you do well

It's human nature to do what comes easiest and what you do best. But it is a dangerous mistake. It leads to muscle imbalances and injury. It also is a very inefficient way to train. How many people do you see in gym doing pull-ups? Maybe one? They are hard. Yet they are the best exercise for your back, core, and biceps. And you won't ever be able to do them unless you start doing them. So leave your ego at the door and go for it. You'll get points from everyone else at the gym just for trying.

Once you are a pro and can do all the exercises in your chapter safely and with perfect form, I want you to take them on to a balance board like a BOSU board. This will add a new dimension of difficulty and stress and strengthen your muscles even more.

A second way to up your intensity is to add a pause during the exercise. For example, pause halfway down during your push-up hold for 2 seconds and then continue the movement. The way to continue to improve is by making changes in your exercise program that continue to stress your muscles. Stay out of your comfort zone and find ways to mix up your exercise routine.

COOLDOWN

The cooldown is important to minimize muscle soreness and fatigue. During exercise, your body accumulates lactic acid (a by-product of muscle work). We associate lactic acid buildup with muscle soreness. The cooldown period gives your body a chance to clear the lactic acid from your muscles and so minimizes postworkout discomfort.

Do not stop exercising abruptly. If you simply stop after exercising vigorously, then there is a good chance your blood pressure will drop and you will get light-headed and dizzy. Keep moving. It's what all the experts say and for very good reason. Especially if you have any history of coronary artery disease, then you need to make the cooldown period an important priority. Think of the cooldown period as "active rest," where you are gently returning your body to its pre-exercise state. Walk slowly for about 10 minutes after you finish exercising to gently return your heart rate to its resting level. Or you can simply do a slower version of whatever exercise you were doing. Continue walking until you are breathing normally and can easily carry on a conversation. Your cooldown period is the best time to stretch. But wait until your heart rate has slowed and is approaching your resting rate. If you suffer joint pain or low back pain, then this is the optimal time to stretch. Your goal is to correct muscle imbalances that contribute to pain and improve your joint range of motion. Your physical therapist can teach you more about this.

And don't forget to rehydrate. Water is the best fluid for rehydration unless you have been exercising at a high intensity for an hour or more. None of us needs the calories of the electrolyte drinks, and rarely do we lose enough salt with routine exercise to require extra salt found in these sport drinks.

There you have it. The basics you need to get started. Now it is up to you. Your life and health is within your control. You *can* do this; I will be your guide.

EXERCISE TO TREAT HYPERTENSION

Here is one area where exercise really makes an impact in the treatment and prevention of disease. A regular exercise program has been recommended by such renowned groups as the World Health Organization to combat high blood pressure and the cardiovascular risk factors that go along with it. And that's one of the biggest problems with hypertension; it's all the other stuff that goes along with it that makes it such a risky disease. In addition to causing strokes and kidney failure, high blood pressure is closely linked with increased risk of heart attack, heart failure, and even death. All you need is to increase your blood pressure from 115/75 to 135/95 mmHg and your risk for heart disease doubles. Doubles. Ouch. That's a little too much risk for my taste. And yet we continue to play with fire. There are over 58 million Americans diagnosed with high blood pressure, and many of them are not well controlled with medication. But clinical trials have shown that exercise can lower blood pressure as much as some drugs. Now couple that with the extra 20 lb. you're going to lose with regular exercise (and diet, of course), and you'll be off meds before you know it. That's amazing; your lifestyle choices are as powerful as any medication prescribed by your physician. Doctors know how important exercise is. They tell every one of their patients to get exercising. But although doctors know a lot about your disease, we don't have a quick, easy answer to your question "So how do I start?" or "What do I do?" Well, here you go. Here is your start. The following is a guided program to start you on a safe and effective program to change your life and treat your disease. So let's get you started on that regular exercise program. It has no side effects like the medications you're taking, only benefits.

WHY EXERCISE?

This is the exciting part. You can see the beneficial effect of exercise after your first exercise session. This is in addition to the generalized decrease in your blood pressure that occurs after weeks of exercise training. The drop in your blood pressure after a bout of exercise is termed post-exercise hypotension. And it can last for up to 22 hours after exercise. See why we recommend daily aerobic exercise for people with high blood pressure? You get immediate results. And the biggest effects are seen in those who need it the most. There is a small drop in blood pressure after exercise in healthy young subjects, but the biggest decrease in blood pressure is seen in those with real hypertension. So as little as one exercise session can significantly drop your blood pressure for the rest of the day. Why not do it every day?

Over 75% of you can bring your blood pressure under control with a regular exercise routine of moderate intensity. You can kiss that little pill bottle good-bye (aren't you taking enough of them already?), kiss all those nasty side effects good-bye, and use the hundreds of dollars you have saved to buy those season football tickets or that designer purse you've been dreaming of. Both the words *moderate* and *regular* are important. Moderate is a good thing. It means that studies have shown that light-to-moderate exercise results in a drop in blood pressure. No need to exercise vigorously—unless you're a glutton for punishment. However, you do have to make a commitment, and you have to stick with it. If you stop exercising, the beneficial effects of exercise reverse back to your pretraining state. So you must make the commitment to exercise on a regular basis, or it's back to the pill bottle.

Exercise is not only important for the treatment of hypertension after you've been diagnosed, but also for the prevention of the disease. You can actually keep yourself from getting high blood pressure by starting a regular exercise program. People who are physically active have a 25%–50% lower risk of developing hypertension. If you are overweight, in poor physical shape, or if high blood pressure runs in your family, then you are at significant risk for developing hypertension, and you need to get moving now. By treating or preventing high blood pressure, you are minimizing your risk for heart disease and every other disease discussed in this book. We know that lack of physical activity is actually a major risk factor for cardiovascular disease and death in middle-aged men and women. Not old, middle-aged.

Lastly, and unfortunately most important in this economic climate, maintaining your health and fitness is a monetary decision. There is less money than ever available for health care. So the sicker you choose to be, the more of your hard-earned dollars are going to pills and doctor visits. Poor choice. Fixable choice. And your choice starts here.

BEFORE YOU BEGIN

I appreciate your caution in starting a program on your own. You're right to be cautious. There are risks when patients with high blood pressure and heart disease exercise, but the risks of not exercising far outweigh the risks of activity. So you don't get to use this as an excuse for not starting. We'll discuss how to get started safely and the things to watch out for while you are exercising.

Before starting any exercise program, you should get clearance from your doctor. Sounds familiar, I know. But it is much more than a way for me to cover my legal behind. Patients with hypertension are known to be at risk for heart disease and should get the OK from their doctor before beginning any vigorous exercise activity. However, if you smoke, are obese, have a blood pressure above 180/110 mmHg, have a history of cardiac disease (e.g., you have had bypass surgery or a heart attack), then you must be evaluated before starting *any* exercise program. Your doctor may want you to have a stress test before starting. In addition, if you have certain symptoms like new or worsening chest pain, shortness of breath, or palpitations, then you should get in to see him soon and wait to start your exercise program until he/she gives you the green light.

We know that regular exercise will help protect you from developing heart disease. But vigorous activity (more than 60% of your maximum) may actually cause a heart attack in a very few selected people. So go see your doctor before you begin a strenuous program to make sure you're not one of those unlucky ones. In addition, if you are a man over the age of 45 or a woman over the age of 50, then it is strongly recommended that you have a stress test before starting an exercise program. These recommendations are from the American College of Sports Medicine based on the prevalence of heart disease in this country. Please check with your doctor. These recommendations are for first-time exercisers. However, while you're waiting for that doctor's appointment, I encourage you to start your walking program. Light activity is the perfect way to start and is not associated with increased cardiac risk. In fact, that is how I will tell you to start your program anyway.

SAFETY PRECAUTIONS FOR PATIENTS WITH HYPERTENSION

There are a few considerations that are unique to hypertension and the medications used to treat it that can influence your exercise routine. You should keep these in mind:

1. If you are taking certain blood pressure medications, beta-blockers, and diuretics, then you need to be especially careful about exercising in the heat. Using these medications makes you more susceptible to heat illness and also a fall in your blood sugar when you exercise in hot or humid environment. So if you are going to exercise in the heat, then you must know the warning signs of heat illness, wear clothing that helps wick away the sweat to keep you cool (no rubber pants, please), exercise during the cooler times of day, and adjust your exercise intensity downward when it is hot outside.

2. Cooldown is especially important if you are currently taking blood pressure medication. Alpha-blockers, calcium channel blockers, and vasodilators can cause an abrupt fall in your blood pressure if you stop exercising suddenly. To prevent a sudden drop in blood pressure (and the fainting that could result), you must gradually cool down by slowly walking for about 10 minutes after your exercise session. If you don't know what kind of blood pressure medication you are taking, then ask your doctor. It's your responsibility to know.

3. Again, if you have severe or uncontrolled hypertension, then you should not start an exercise program until after you have been cleared by your physician and they have started you on or adjusted your medications to better control your blood pressure.

4. Remember that calcium channel blockers and beta-blockers (two medications used to treat heart disease and hypertension) will blunt your heart rate's response to exercise. You may

be working very hard, but your heart rate is still in the lazy zone according to your heart rate monitor. For you, heart rate is not a good indicator of your exercise intensity. Leave the monitor at home. Instead, I recommend using your breathing rate and how hard you feel you are working to guide your exercise intensity rather than a heart rate monitor (refer to chapter 2).

5. And lastly, if you take blood pressure or heart medication, the timing of your exercise program is important. You don't want an exercise to block absorption of your medications. Moderate-intensity exercise should be delayed for about 3 hours after taking your pills so that they are fully absorbed from your gut. With moderate- to-high-intensity exercise, blood is shunted away from your stomach and directed to your working muscles. So wait several hours after taking your medication before you start to exercise seriously. There should be no problem with a light walk right after you take your pills. The safe window is exercising 3–10 hours after your take your medication. That way your medications will have their full protective effect during your exercise session.

LET'S GET STARTED: YOUR EXERCISE PROGRAM

As we've discussed, a well-rounded exercise program includes four components: aerobic exercise, strength training, balance, and flexibility. Regardless of your disease and fitness level, each of these should be part of your exercise routine. But because you have high blood pressure, I have modified each of these components to meet the specific treatment goals and limitations imposed by your disease. Since you have hypertension, the focus of your exercise program will be on lowering your blood pressure, heart health, and weight loss. If your exercise time is limited, then put your time into aerobics. Here is the outline of your exercise program:

Warm-up for 10 minutes before starting each exercise session.

Aerobic exercise for 10 minutes 3 days a week initially, then progress to 30 minutes 5–6 days a week over the next 2–3 months. Start at an intensity of 4–5 on the Borg scale if you are new to exercise and work up to an intensity that is 60%–70% of your max (6–7 on the Borg scale).

Resistance training for 15 minutes 3 days a week to supplement your aerobic work. Do 15–20 reps of each exercise using lighter weights. And breathe with every movement to avoid dangerous increases in your blood pressure.

Cooldown for 10 minutes after each session.

These are your guidelines. The most important thing you can do is learn to listen to your body and adapt how hard and how long you exercise to its needs. If your knees are hurting during exercise and continue to hurt for several hours after you're done, then that is a signal that you pushed too hard and need to slow down the next session. If you are no longer winded during your exercise session, then that is a signal that your body is getting stronger and you need to pick up your pace to provide a continuous exercise challenge. If you are exercising and just don't have the energy or the drive to continue, then listen to your body and stop for the day. Pat yourself on the back for the work that you have done and go home. You can work harder the next time. Remember, you don't have to be an aerobic animal every day to make significant progress. But you do need to listen to your body and respect what it is telling you. That is especially true if you have heart disease and high blood pressure. On the flip side, if you can't find the motivation to get started, then just tell yourself to go for a 10-minute walk. Just get yourself off the couch and move. I'll bet once you get going, your walk time turns from 10 minutes to 30 minutes. But if it doesn't, then still pat yourself on the back for taking a positive step for your health.

WARM-UP (5-10 minutes before every exercise session)

Three hours after taking your heart medications, you will start with a slow walk and gradually increase your pace over the next 5–10 minutes until your body has slowly and carefully warmed up. Your goal is to increase your pace gradually until you are working at a 5/10 on the Borg scale. At the end of your warm-up phase, your body literally feels warm, and you are breathing heavily. Now you are ready to begin your aerobic work. Your warm-up and cooldown are especially important to ease your heart into and out of the demands of exercise.

AEROBIC EXERCISE (30 minutes 5–6 days a week)

So you have been cleared by your doctor to start an exercise program. And in all his wisdom, he recommends starting with a walking program. I agree 100%. How hard should you exercise, and what intensity is safe if you have high blood pressure? Anyone who is sedentary and beginning an exercise program for the first time should start at a very low intensity (40%–50% maximum or a perceived exertion of 4–5) and gradually increase your effort as tolerated. Start with just 10–15 minutes of exercise a day. Do this 3–4 times a week. To start.

If you have been exercising on a regular basis and are using this book to get smarter and more efficient about what you do, then you should start with 30 minutes of aerobic work. Your goal for blood pressure control is eventually 30–40 minutes per day at an exertion level of 5–7 on the perceived exertion scale. And you should schedule this most days of the week. Make your exercise session a scheduled part of your workweek and put it on your calendar just like you do all your important appointments. Because a single bout of exercise can lower your blood pressure for 22–23 hours after exercise, it only makes sense to take advantage of this at least 5 days a week. By making this regular commitment, you will find that the amount or number of blood pressure medications you need to take will decrease. You may be able to stop your meds completely. And if excess body fat is adding or contributing to your elevated blood pressure and high cholesterol (and I promise you that it is), then exercising 5–6 days a week for 30–40 minutes is necessary to burn off that stored fat. You must realize, it took you time to put that fat on and it will take a time commitment to burn it all off.

RESISTANCE EXERCISE (15 minutes 3 days a week)

Resistance exercise or weight training was previously thought to be potentially dangerous for people with heart disease and hypertension. Now we know that isn't true. In fact, it is an important part of your exercise program for strengthening all the muscles in your body including your heart. By improving your muscle strength in the rest of your body, you actually lessen the stress on your heart.

The important thing about exercising with hypertension is not what you do but how you do it. Your exercise program should consist primarily of aerobic exercise with some resistance training thrown in for good measure. There is no reason that you can't lift weights with high blood pressure, but there are certain precautions. Use weights that you guess to be about one-half as heavy as the maximum amount of weight you can lift. Each set should be 15–20 repetitions. That means you should find a weight that is light enough that you can easily do 15 repetitions with perfect form. But it also needs to be heavy enough so that by rep 20 you feel like you've been working. Avoid lifting very heavy weights and make sure you exhale every time you move the weight. This will help you avoid the Valsalva maneuver (when you strain hard while holding your breath). Many gym rats think that holding their breath helps them to lift more weight, but instead, it dangerously elevates their blood pressure. You cannot be the guy or gal at the gym grunting and groaning against too heavy a weight. It's low weights and many reps for you.

Because you don't have any pain limitations, I have selected some of my favorite exercises for you. These exercises are designed to use a number of muscle groups at a time to optimize the efficiency of your weight training session so you have more time for cardio work. Select one or two exercises from each group to provide a complete full-body workout. Additional exercises are given so you can change your routine every 4–6 weeks. This change will continue to challenge your body and keep you from reaching a plateau.

You can do anything as long as you remember the rule. Low weights, lots of reps.

LEGS AND GLUTES

Pick one exercise from each of the leg sections: glutes, hamstrings, and calves. The exercises in these sections have good overlap, so you'll be working the same muscles several ways, just with a different focus in each grouping. Start with just one exercise per group and later increase the number to continue to challenge your muscles. Pick new exercises every 4–6 weeks. And don't forget the balance exercises at the end of this section.

LEGS–QUADS

Step Up

Stand straight with your stomach strong. Step your right foot onto first step and slowly straighten leg. Keep toes facing front. Bring left foot up to touch step by right ankle, then slowly lower your weight to count of 4 onto left leg. Don't push off back leg. Move slowly so the muscles, and not the momentum, do the work. As you stand up, press your weight through the heel, not the ball, of your foot. Repeat 10-15 times on each leg. When the stair step becomes easy, carry 5–10 lb. dumbbells to increase difficulty; just keep breathing. (Targets quadriceps and glutes, balance).

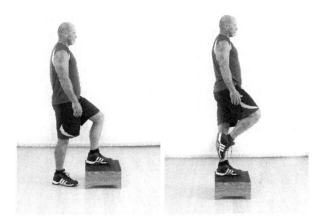

Sit to Stand

Sit on a firm straight-backed chair. Engage your core (tighten your stomach like someone was going to punch you in the gut). With stomach strong, slowly stand up. Use your legs, not your arms, to lift your body off the chair. If you cannot stand without using your arms, then allow them to assist you—but no more than necessary. Slowly lower back to the seated position, but halfway down, pause for a count of 2 or 4, then continue to the seated position. Do as many as you can, maintaining perfect form times. (Targets quadriceps, core).

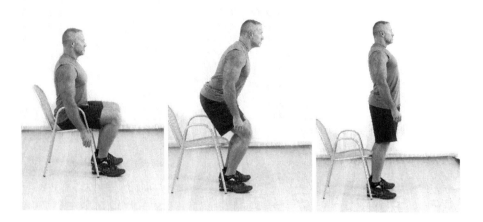

Hip Abduction

Stand facing a chair. With your arms on the back of a chair for balance, slowly raise your right leg out to the side and hold for a count of 2. Lower and repeat with the left leg. As it gets easy, increase the height you lift your leg, and don't hold on. Work up to 12 reps on each side (targets hip abductors, balance).

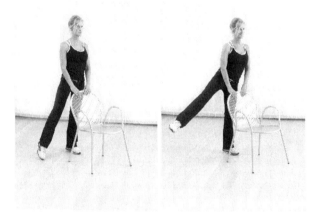

Wall Squat

Stand with a fitness ball between you and a wall. Rest your lower back against the fitness ball. Your feet should be shoulder width apart and about 3 feet away from the wall. Slowly bend your knees till your thighs are parallel to the floor or as low as you can go. Make sure you keep your knees directly over your toes. Pause and then squeeze your buttocks as you return to the standing position. Build up to 15-20 reps. As this gets easy, deepen your knee bend to optimize quad strengthening (targets quadriceps, glutes).

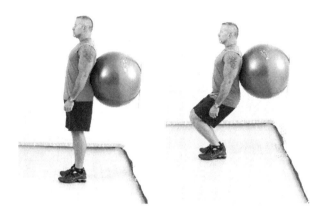

Fitness Ball Single-Leg Squat

Stand facing away from a fitness ball, about 2 feet in front of it. Place your right foot on the ball. With your weight on your left leg, bend your left knee and let your right leg roll back on the ball. Keep your left knee straight over your toes. Pause and return to a stand. Build to 12–15 repetitions with each leg. When this gets easy, hold 3 or 5 lb. dumbbells in your hands (targets quads and glutes, balance).

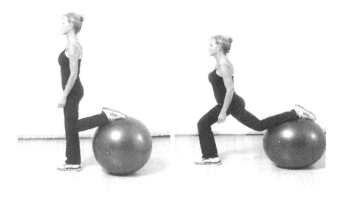

Sumo Squat

Stand with your feet more than shoulder width apart and toes pointed out to the sides at a 45-degree angle. Hold a 3–5 lb. dumbbell with both hands and let your arms hang straight down. Slowly bend your knees, all the while keeping your knees out over your toes. Use weights that let you easily do 15 reps while maintaining perfect form (targets glutes, quads, and inner thighs).

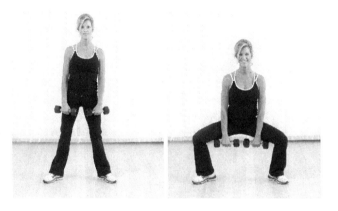

LEGS–HAMSTRINGS

Pick one of these exercises to start with. Change every 4–6 weeks.

Dumbbell Leg Curl

Lie facedown on a bench and have your workout partner place a light dumbbell between your feet with one end of the dumbbell resting on the soles of your shoes. Bend your knees and bring your feet toward your buttocks. Hold the dumbbell tight between your feet. Keep your hips flat on the bench. Pause and then lower the weight to the starting position. Do 15–20 reps (targets hamstrings and glutes).

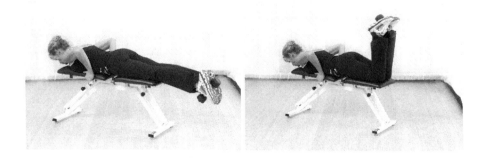

Hip Bridge

Lying on your back with heels tucked close to your buttocks, lift your buttocks off the ground so your body forms a straight line from knees to shoulders. Hold for 2 seconds, then slowly lower over a 2-second count. Do 15-20 reps (targets hamstrings, glutes, and low back).

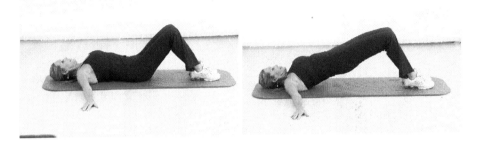

For added difficulty, straighten your right leg from the knee and do the movement using only the left leg to lift your body. Keep the right leg straight during the exercise. Do 15–20 reps on each side.

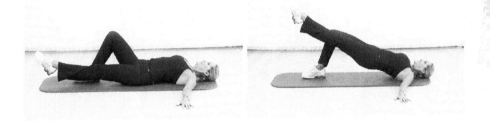

For even more difficulty, straighten your right leg with your toes pointing at the ceiling. Keep your leg pointed toward the ceiling as you raise your body with your left leg. Do 15–20 reps, then repeat with the left leg straight.

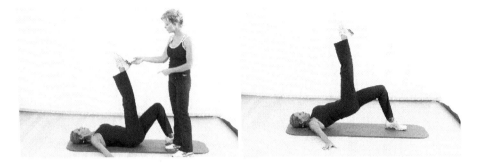

Fire Hydrant

Kneel on all fours on a mat and place a 1 or 3 lb. weight behind your right knee. Squeeze your leg muscles so that the dumbbell stays locked in place. Keeping your back flat and your head down, slowly raise your right leg until your thigh is parallel with the floor. Pause and then lower your right leg to the starting position. Do 15–20 reps with each leg (targets hamstrings and glutes).

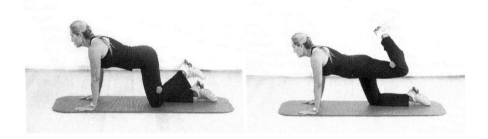

LEGS–CALVES

Pick one of these exercises to start with. Change every 4–6 weeks.

Seated Calf Raise

Sit with 5 or 10 lb. dumbbells resting on each knee. Slowly lift your knees and come up on the balls of your feet. Pause for a count of 2 and then slowly lower. Make sure that you're using your calves to raise the weights and not your arms. Repeat 15–20 times (targets calves).

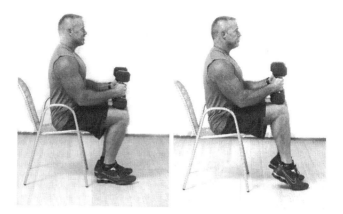

Standing Calf Raise

Stand on a step or a block with the toes and ball of your right foot at the edge of the step. Hold on to a wall or chair with your left hand for balance. Cross your left foot behind your right ankle and balance yourself on the ball of your right foot. Lower your heel as far as you can until you feel a stretch in the back of your calf. Lift your heel as high as you can, pause, and return to the starting position. Do 10–15 reps and repeat with the left leg (targets calves, balance).

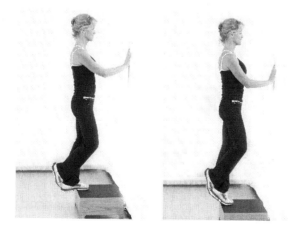

BALANCE

Pick 2 exercises from the following group and change exercises every 4–6 weeks.

Eyes Closed

Stand on a thick folded towel with your feet shoulder width apart. Stand tall with your abdominal muscles engaged (say *sshhh* to engage them). Close your eyes and visualize the upright position.

Balance on One Leg

Stand with your hand on a chair or bar for support. Shift your weight to your left leg and lift the right leg off the floor. Try letting go of your support or only resting your fingertips on the bar for balance. Your goal is to stand on one leg for 30 seconds. Turn around and repeat it standing on your right leg.

Advanced

Fold a bath towel several times over, place it on the floor, and stand on the center of the towel. This will give you a slightly unstable surface because the towel is soft.

Advanced

Try doing the one-leg balance with your eyes shut. Keep the chair back close so you can steady yourself as needed.

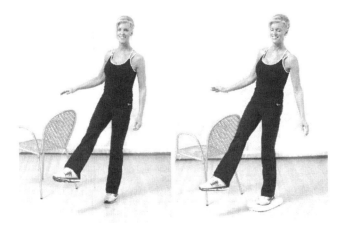

Toe-Stand Balance

Stand facing a sturdy chair or bar with your hands resting lightly on it. Rise up onto your toes and try to let go of the chair and balance for a count of 10. When you are an expert, raise up on your toes and, still holding on gently, shift your weight to the right leg, and try to balance on your toes on one leg. You will feel the muscles of your entire leg and your core engage. Keep your head high and stomach strong (say *sshhh*).

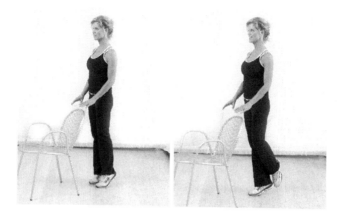

Lunge with Trunk Rotation

Stand with your right leg one stride in front of the left with the left heel lifted, abdominals tensed, and your arms out at your side at shoulder height. Bend both knees and lower your hips directly between the two legs so your right thigh is parallel with the floor. Make sure your knees are in line with your toes. Use your hip and thigh muscles to bring your left leg through and forward till the left knee is at hip level. As you raise your left leg, twist your body so you look over your left thigh. Return to the starting position and repeat 8 times. If you can. This is a very tough exercise when done correctly. Then alternate legs and repeat with the right leg (targets quadriceps, hamstrings, glutes, calves, abdominals, and lower back).

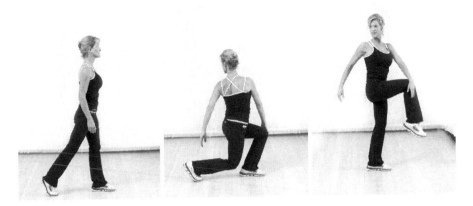

CORE

Although you'll see everyone in the gym dropping to do 50 sit-ups to strengthen their core, they are defeating the purpose on several fronts. The first problem is the number 50. Any exercise you do where you can do more than 20 is not building strength efficiently. Your best bet is to slow down the exercise so you recruit more muscle fibers and build strength efficiently. Doing 50 sit-ups does not provide enough muscle resistance to build strength. Working your abs slowly or adding weight will recruit the maximal number of muscle fibers and provide optimal strength gains. Find 1 or 2 exercises that are hard enough that you can only do 15–20 reps. Just don't forget to breathe. It's extra hard to remember to breathe when you're working your abs.

The second problem is with the word *sit-up*. It's a bad choice of an exercise to build core strength. You see, any exercise where you raise your body up from the floor is using your hip flexor muscles far more than it uses your abdominal muscles. So with the classic sit-up, you are training your hip flexors but not your abdominal/core muscles. The sit-up is not only ineffective, but it is also potentially dangerous. It can easily strain your low back, a situation we want to avoid. The exercises that follow are safe for your back and will develop all four of your abdominal muscles, providing the strong core you need. Your core muscles include your rectus abdominis muscle, which is your six-pack. But there are three other sets of muscles that run underneath the rectus muscles. These three sets of muscles run diagonally and across your belly and are the ones we want to strengthen. The following exercises focus on strengthening these. Core also includes your low back muscles. They work in tandem with your abdominal muscles to provide support for your back. Pick a combination of exercises from the list below that work both.

You should do 2–3 of the following exercises as part of your weight training program. After 4–6 weeks, switch exercises.

Medicine Ball Twist

Sit on the floor with your legs extended and your back straight. Place a medicine ball (start with a light ball) next to your right hip. Twist and pick up the ball and place it beside the opposite hip. Repeat on each side for a total of 12–15 reps.

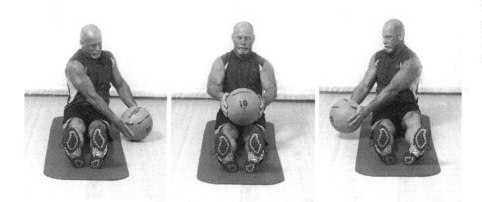

Resistance One-Leg Crunch

Lie on your back with your knees bent with your feet on the floor. Lift your right knee and resist the movement with your right arm. Hold for a count of 2 and then return to the starting position. Repeat on the left. That is 1 repetition. Work up so you can do 12–15 reps (targets abs).

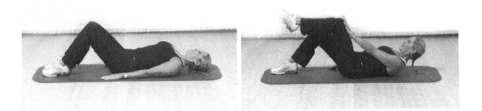

Plank

This is one of my favorite core-strengthening exercises.

Assume a modified push-up position with your forearms resting on the floor. Elbows should be under your shoulders and bent at 90 degrees. Keep your torso steady and your body in a straight line from your head to your toes. Do not let your stomach sag. Hold for as long as you can. Your goal is to hold this for 30 seconds (targets core-stabilizing muscles).

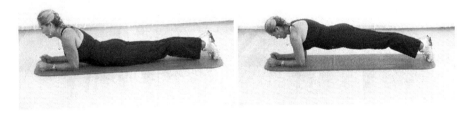

Cable (or Dumbbell) Woodchopper

Stand with your right side toward the weight stack of a cable machine. Grab the rope handle of a high pulley with both hands. Pull the cable across your body until your hands are across your body just outside your left knee. Slowly reverse the move to return to the starting position (targets abs, shoulders, back, and legs).

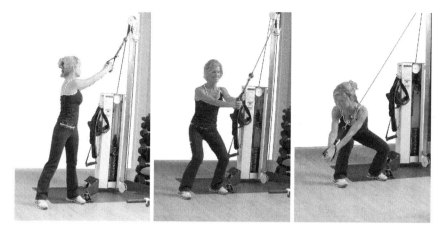

To Use Dumbbells

Hold light dumbbell with hand over handgrip with your arms extended above your right shoulder. Keep your arms straight but don't lock your elbows. Bend your knees and lower the weight down and across your body until your hands reach the outside of your left ankle. Pause then quickly reverse the movement pausing at the top. That is 1 repetition. Use a weight that is light enough that you can do 15–20 repetitions.

Reverse Cable Woodchopper

Now attach the rope handle to the low pulley cable. Bend over and grab the rope with both hands. Your arms should be nearly straight and just outside your right knee. Keeping your arms straight, pull the rope up across your body until your hands are in line with your left ear. Slowly reverse the movement and return to your original position in a controlled manner. Do 15–20 reps (targets abdominals, shoulders, back, and legs).

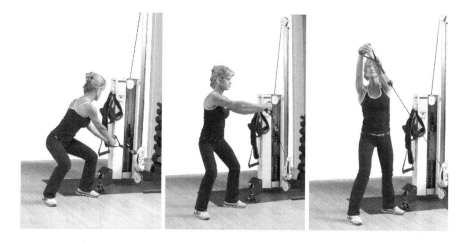

To Use Dumbbells

Crouch down using a light dumbbell with hand over handgrip with your arms extended beside your right bent knee. Keep your arms straight but don't lock your elbows. Straighten your knees as you lift the weight across your body until your hands are raised over your head past your left shoulder. Pause then slowly lower the weight back to the starting position. That is 1 repetition. Use a weight that is light enough that you can do 15–20 repetitions on each side.

Dryland Swimming

Lie on your stomach on an exercise pad (you might want a towel under your hips for comfort) with your arms extended overhead. Lift your arms and legs off the floor at the same time so they are about 6–8 inches off the ground. Keep looking at the floor. Kick your legs up and down like you are swimming. While you are kicking, move your arms from above your head to your sides and back over your head. Kick for as long as you can, avoiding soreness in your low back (targets back, glutes, and legs).

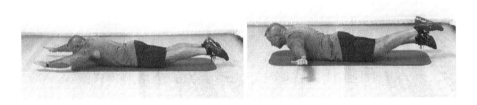

Suitcase Walk

Hold a 3 or 5 lb. dumbbell in your right hand at your side. Keeping your body in perfect alignment, walk as far as you can without discomfort. Repeat with the dumbbell in the other hand. Walk progressively longer distances to challenge your core. Stand tall with stomach strong and shoulders back. Remember to check yourself by saying *sshhh*. This will engage your core the correct way. Increase the amount of weight you carry as the exercise gets easier (targets core-stabilizing muscles).

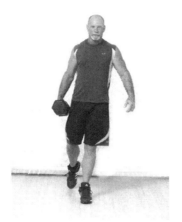

Prone Hip Extension

Lie facedown over a bench or padded stool with your legs hanging off the edge. Tighten/engage your abs and lift both legs to hip height so you form a straight line with your body. Hold for a count of 5, then slowly lower. Repeat 10–15 times.

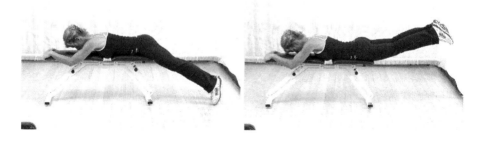

Bicycle

Lie on your back and lift your legs straight in the air. Keep your hands on your stomach to make sure it stays strong and your back stays flat on the floor. Move your legs like you are pedaling a bike. Do this for 30 seconds (targets abs).

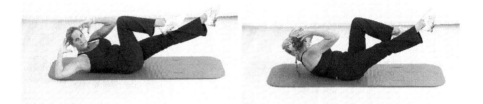

Superman

This works your back extensor muscles with minimal stress on your spine compared to more traditional back exercises. Kneel on your hands and knees. Keep your stomach tight (like you're being punched) but keep the normal arch in your lower back. Straighten your right leg behind you, keeping it at hip level. Then raise your right arm so it extends straight out at ear level. Keep both your outstretched arm and leg parallel to the floor. Hold for a count of 4, then repeat on the other side. Do 12–15 repetitions each side (targets lower back, glutes, and hamstrings).

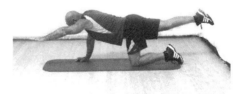

When that becomes simple, start from a standard push-up position and raise your left leg while maintaining the perfect push-up position. Repeat with the left leg. Hold as long as you can (targets abdominals, back, hamstrings, and glutes).

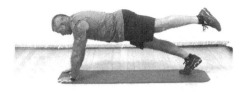

BACK

This section supplements the lower back work found in the core section with upper back work. This should be one of your target spots to fight the shoulder slump of old age. You can combat the humped posture with a strong back and a good balance between chest and upper back strength. In other words, don't overdo your chest work just because it is an area you can see and admire. What your admirers really love is good posture and squared-off shoulders. Pick 1–2 exercises from this section and select a new exercise every 4–6 weeks.

Wall Slide

Stand with your buttocks, upper back, and head against the wall. Raise your arms over your head so your shoulders, elbows, and wrists also touch the wall. Maintaining these points of contact, bend your arms until your elbows are tucked in at your sides. You should feel a contraction in your shoulders and the muscles between your shoulder blades. Reverse the move. Do 12–15 reps (targets upper back).

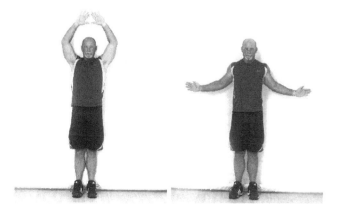

Classic Row Revisited

Sit at the rowing station with your knees bent and your back straight. This will be a much smaller movement that the classic row but you will get the same upper back strengthening benefit. Squeeze your shoulder blades together, and in a count of 2, bring the handles to your chest. Keep your shoulder blades squeezed together as you slowly straighten your arms. Do 15–20 reps (targets upper back).

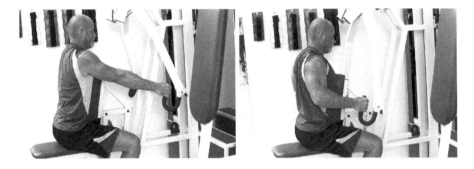

Dumbbell Single-Arm Row

Holding a dumbbell in your right hand, place your left knee and left hand on a bench. Your right arm should be straight and hang just in front of your shoulder. Keeping your back flat and right elbow close to your body, pull the dumbbell up and back toward your hip. Pause and then slowly lower the weight. Repeat 15–20 times, then switch sides (targets upper back).

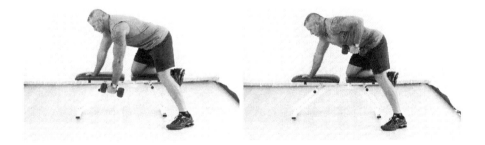

Dumbbell Row with Rotation

Stand with your feet shoulder width apart and hold a 1 or 3 lb. dumbbell in each hand. Bend forward at the waist. Keep your back flat and your core strong. Bend your knees and let the dumbbells hang in front of your thighs, palms facing each other. Start by pulling your right arm up to your rib cage while rotating your shoulders and torso as far as you can to the right. Pause and then slowly lower your right arm while pulling your left arm up to your chest and rotating your body to the left. Remember to keep your core rock-hard strong during the entire exercise. Do 15–20 reps each side (targets upper back and core).

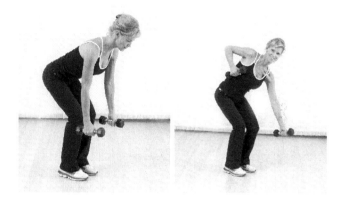

Lat Pull Down

Sit at the lat pull-down station. Adjust the leg pads so your legs fit secure underneath. Grab the bar and begin by pulling your shoulder blades down and together. Keep them pinched tight and then pull the bar down toward the floor (or if you are using a bar, then pull it down to chest height). Keep your back straight and move slowly through the full range of motion. Do 15–20 reps (targets back).

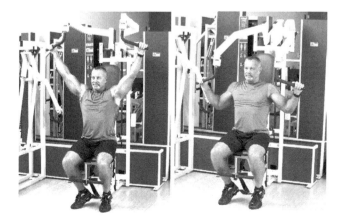

Fitness Ball Y

Lie on a fitness ball with your legs straight and your chest off the ball. Let your fists rest on the floor with your arms hanging down in front of your shoulders. Lift your arms up and to the sides, forming at 45-degree angles to form a Y. While you are raising your arms, focus on moving your shoulder blades back and down. Reverse the move back to the starting position. When you can repeat this 15–20 times, then do it holding 1–3 lb. weights (targets back).

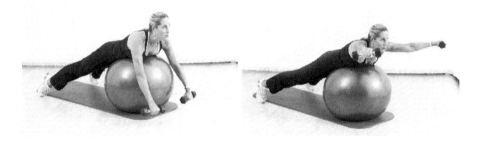

Fitness Ball T

Lie on a fitness ball with your legs straight and your chest off the ball. Let your hands rest on the floor with your arms straight. Squeeze your shoulder blades together and raise your arms straight out to the sides, forming a T with your torso and arms. Reverse the move back to the starting position. When you can repeat this 15–20 times, then do it holding 1–3 lb. weights (targets back).

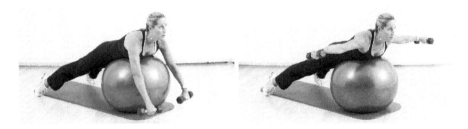

SHOULDERS

Pick one of these exercises to start with. Change every 4–6 weeks.

Shoulder Shrug

Stand holding a 3–5 lb. dumbbell in each hand, palms facing toward each other. Shrug your shoulders up to your ears and pause. Slowly lower your shoulders. Repeat 15–20 times (targets shoulders).

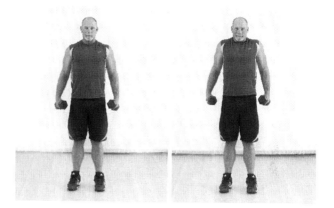

Shoulder Raise

Sit on a bench holding a 1 or 3 lb. weight. Raise the weight out to the side until your arm is at a 90-degree angle at the shoulder. Slowly bring the weight to the front, keeping your arm at the same 90-degree height. Repeat on the other side. Do 15–20 reps each side. When your shoulder feels stable with the 1 lb. weight, you can step up to a heavier weight. You can also do this exercise standing to engage your core muscles for a double benefit (targets shoulders).

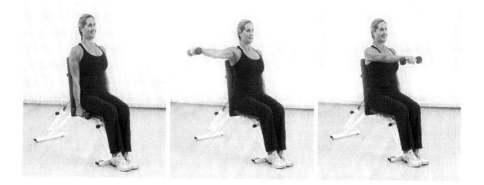

Controlled Fly

Kneel on a bench with your right leg and right arm on the bench. In your left hand, you are holding a 1 or 3 lb. weight with the palm facing you. Keep your back flat and stomach strong during the exercise. Slowly lift the weight out to the side till your arm is parallel to the floor. Do 15–20 reps with each arm (targets shoulders).

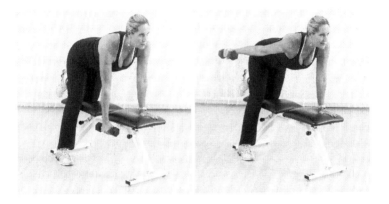

Toss and Catch

Play toss and catch with a beach ball or light medicine ball. As the exercise gets easier, you can increase the weight of the ball. Keep your stomach engaged (tense the muscles like you're going to be punched in the stomach) throughout your game, especially right before you throw the ball (targets shoulders and abs).

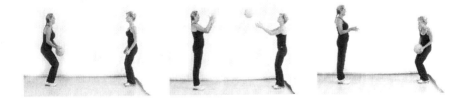

Alternating Shoulder Dumbbell Press

By alternating your arms, you also get core strengthening with the exercise.

Sit with your back supported. Engage your core (like you are preparing to be punched). This will provide a solid core to protect your back and double the value of the exercise by working your stomach muscles. Hold a 1–3 lb. dumbbell in each hand at shoulder level with palms facing each other. Press the dumbbell in your right hand straight above you until your arm is straight and the weight is above your head. Then slowly lower the weight to the starting position. Repeat on the left. Do a total of 8–12 per side (targets shoulders and core).

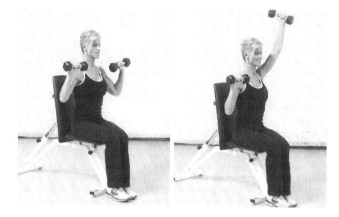

Advanced

Do the same exercise standing or stand on one leg to challenge your core. Keep your abdominal muscles engaged.

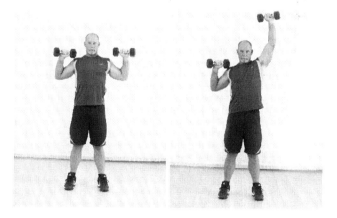

CHEST

Pick one of these exercises to start with. Change every 4–6 weeks.

Wall Push-ups (the perfect beginner's exercise)

Stand at arm's length from the wall. Put both hands on the wall at chest level. Slowly bend your elbows to the count of 4 and then slowly straighten them. Repeat 12 times. When this is easy, go to the modified push-up below (targets chest).

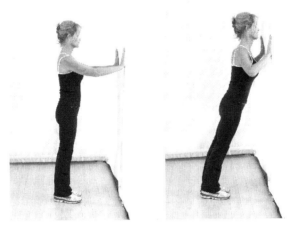

Single-Arm Bench Press

Lie on your back on a bench holding a dumbbell in your right hand next to your chest with your palm facing you. Keep your left arm beside you for balance. Push the dumbbell up so your arm is straight above your chest. Pause then slowly lower the weight to the starting position. Alternate arms and use a weight you can easily control for 15–20 reps on each side (targets chest).

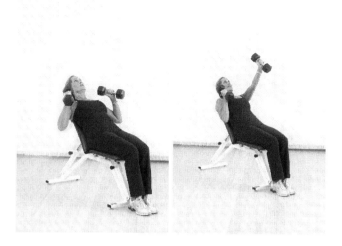

Push-ups on Knees

I know these are girl push-ups, but done correctly, they will result in impressive improvements in your strength. Once you can do 12 of these with perfect form, then it is time to do them in the regular push-up position. Keep your core strong throughout the push-up by maintaining a straight line from your knees to the top of your head.

Kneel on the floor with your knees on a pad. Walk your arms out until your body is in a straight line with your knees bent. In this modified push-up position, I want you to slowly lower your body (keeping a straight line from the tip of your head to your knees) until you are barely touching the floor and then slowly return to the starting position, keeping perfect form (targets chest).

Do 6–12 reps in each of the three-hand positions illustrated.

A) Normal push-up position—elbows are at a 90-degree angle with your hands right under your elbows.

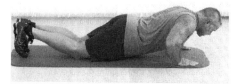

B) Wide-arm position—hands are placed out past your elbows so the angle of your elbows is about 120 degrees.

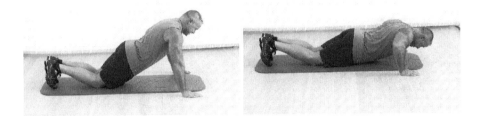

C) Diamond—place your hands so that your thumb and index fingers touch each other and make the shape of a diamond.

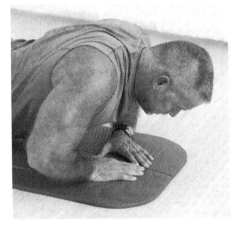

Dumbbell Incline Fly

Lie faceup on an incline bench. Hold 3–5 lb. dumbbells straight over your chest with your palms facing each other. Slowly open your arms, keeping your hands in line with your shoulders. Stop when the weights are level with your chest. Pause and return to the starting position. Repeat 15–20 times (targets chest).

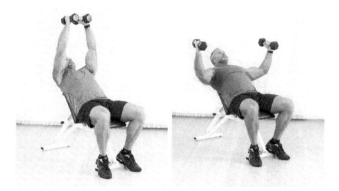

COOLDOWN (10-15 minutes after every exercise session)

Your cooldown is as important as the warm-up phase of your exercise program if you have heart disease and/or hypertension. Do not stop exercising abruptly. If you simply stop after exercising vigorously, then there is a good chance your blood pressure will drop and you will get light-headed and dizzy. Keep moving. It's what all the experts say and for very good reason. Think of the cooldown period as "active rest," where you are gently returning your body to its pre-exercise state. Walk slowly for about 10 minutes after you finish exercising to gently return your heart rate to its resting level. Or you can simply do a slower version of whatever exercise you were doing. Continue walking until you are breathing normally and can easily carry on a conversation. The cooldown period is also important to minimize muscle soreness and fatigue. During exercise, your body accumulates lactic acid (a by-product of muscle work). We associate lactic acid buildup with muscle soreness. The cooldown period gives your body a chance to clear the lactic acid from your muscles, so it minimizes post workout discomfort. Only after your breathing and heart rate have returned to resting levels is it time to stretch.

GENERAL STRETCHES FOR YOUR COOLDOWN

Maintaining flexibility of your muscles will increase your range of motion and provide agility. It is also important to minimize injury. The most important and permanent way to increase your flexibility is to do every exercise you do through the full range of movement. Exercises like lunges, squats, and even push-ups should be done by moving your body through its full pain-free range of motion. As you move your body as far as it can, make sure you keep good form during every repetition. But because they feel so good, I have included my favorite stretches. When you do these stretches, start slowly, breathe deeply, and push just to the limit of pain. You will find that as your joint warms up, you will be able to go a little farther each time. Use your breath to help you relax into each stretch. Take a slow, deep breath in through your nose and then relax into the stretch as you exhale through your mouth. Think about your breath and consciously breathe deep in through your nose, filling your lungs down to their bases. This will help you relax and make the most of each stretch. Bouncing or forcing the stretch is actually counterproductive. *Do not bounce.* Plan to do the majority of your stretching program while you are cooling down—while your muscles are still warm from your exercise session.

Kneeling Quad Stretch

Kneel with your right leg bent in front of you with your knee at a 90-degree angle and your left knee on a mat for cushioning. Keep your body vertical and gently press your hips forward to feel a stretch in the front of the left thigh and hip. Hold for a count of 10, then relax. Repeat 5–10 times and then repeat on the other side.

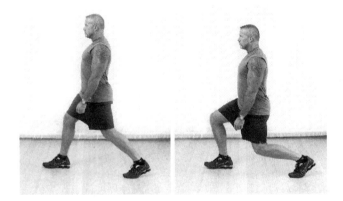

Quadriceps Standing Stretch

Stand facing a chair, holding on to the back lightly for balance. Bend the right knee and grab your ankle with your right hand. Hold for a count of 5, exhaling during the stretch. Try to balance by lifting your hands off the back of the chair on during the stretch to engage core strengthening.

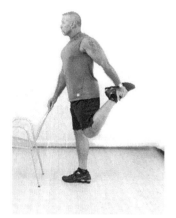

Piriformis Stretch

Lying on your back, bend your right knee with your knee at a 90-degree angle and your foot on the floor. Rest your left ankle on your right leg, and let your knee relax out to the side. Gently pull your right knee to your chest and feel the stretch in the left buttock. Hold for a count of 5, exhaling during the stretch.

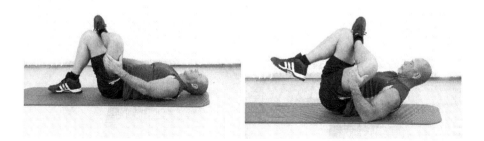

Lying Hamstring Stretch

Lie on your back with both legs straight on the floor and arms by your sides. Bring your right knee to your chest. Place both hands behind your right knee and slowly straighten your right leg. It is OK if you need to lower your right leg to get your knee straight. Hold the straight-leg position for a count of 5, slowly exhaling while you straighten it. Bend the knee again and repeat the exercise 5–10 times on each side.

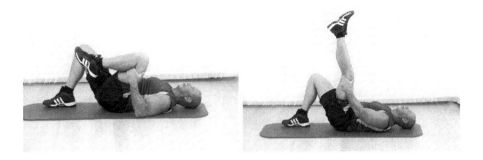

Calf Stretch

Stand on a bottom stair, holding on to the railing for support. Edge your feet back so your heels are off the step. Slowly rise up on your toes and hold for a count of 2. Then lower your body, keeping your knees straight until your heels are below the step and you feel a stretch up the back of your leg.

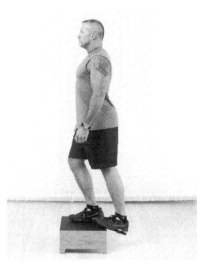

Floor Chest Stretch

Lie faceup on a foam roll with your head supported. Extend your arms out to your sides with your palms facing the ceiling. You will feel a stretch across your chest. Take slow, easy breaths and hold the stretch for 30 seconds. Repeat 3 times.

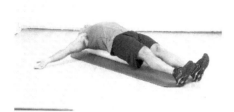

Supine Tuck and Curl

Lie flat on your back, knees bent and feet on the floor. Moving slowly, tilt your pelvis and lift your hips off the floor slightly, then lower. Do 6 reps.

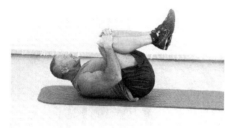

Knee-to-Chest Pose

Lie on your back with your legs fully extended. Draw one knee to your chest and hold it with both hands. Breathe in, and as you breathe out, pull your knee to your chest. Hold for 3–5 breaths. Switch legs and repeat.

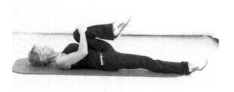

Trunk Twister

Lie on your back on the floor with your arms extended out at shoulder level. Raise your right leg until your toes point to the ceiling. Keeping your leg straight and your shoulders glued to the floor, slowly lower your leg across your body until your toe touches the floor on the left side of your body. Pause at the point that your shoulder wants to lift off the floor. Raise your leg back up in the air and then lower it to the floor. Repeat with your left leg. Do 5–10 repetitions on each side.

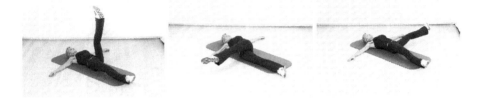

Side Stretch

Stand with your feet apart and stretch your arms over your head as you inhale. Draw a big circle with the fingertips of your right hand as you exhale through your mouth and reach to the side. Hold for a count of two and as you inhale and return to the upright position. Exhale and lower your arms to your sides. Repeat for a total of 8 on each side. This is a very relaxing way to finish your exercise session.

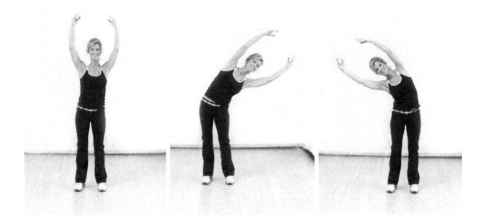

I believe the wise men who say that we are masters of our own fate. Our life is ours, our health is ours, our happiness is ours. Once you take responsibility for your health, you have the power to change it. Stop blaming, stop complaining, and slowly, with love and tenderness, pick yourself up off the couch and go for your first walk. It is the walk of your lifetime.

EXERCISE TO TREAT HEART DISEASE

It is as simple as this. A sedentary lifestyle is one of the major risk factors for heart disease. And heart disease is the leading killer of men and women in America today. In fact, if you're an American male over age 45 or an American female over age 50, then you should just assume that you have some amount of heart disease already present—even if you feel spectacular. Stay active and you simply remove one of the major risk factors (a sedentary lifestyle) from your risk factor profile. Stress and anxiety are other risk factors for heart disease that are also addressed with a regular exercise program. Add in to that the positive effects regular exercise has on hypertension, diabetes, and obesity, and you can do nothing but win by bringing exercise into your life. And you can safely exercise even if you have heart disease, if you follow my direction.

Doctors know how important exercise is. They tell every one of their patients to get exercising. But although doctors know a lot about your disease, we don't have a quick, easy answer to your question "So how do I start?" or "What do I do?" Well, here you go. Here is your start. The following is a guided program to start you on a safe and effective program to change your life and treat your disease.

WHY EXERCISE?

Your heart is a muscle just like your biceps and triceps. And like any other muscle, it gets stronger with exercise. Normally we think of stress as bad, but the stress of exercise is a very positive thing; it results in a stronger, more efficient heart. Exercise also improves the ability of your arteries and veins to circulate blood through your body. Exercise physiologists talk of functional capacity (or your maximal ability to exercise). It refers to your ability to carry out your daily activities with ease. Exercise—by strengthening your heart, blood vessels, and all your muscles—is the only thing that can increase your functional capacity. Sedentary deconditioned individuals have a very low functional capacity, so simple activities like carrying groceries become a major ordeal. The higher your functional capacity, the more reserve you have and the easier your body can tolerate not only the stress of life, but also the stress of illness as well. Every surgeon and anesthesiologist will tell you that the patients who sail easily through surgery are the ones who are physically active on a regular basis. They have a high functional capacity. Their bodies have a reserve to help them recover faster than their sedentary counterparts. In addition, the higher your functional capacity (which is only improved with exercise), the easier it is to climb stairs without being short of breath or work in the garden without getting too tired. In other words, the more fit you are, the easier it is to live your life. There is no medicine or magic food that will make you tougher or stronger. The only way is through exercise.

Exercise by strengthening your heart, lungs, and circulatory system will let you live your life with all the vigor and enthusiasm you want. You will be able to do all the things you want to with ease and still have reserve to enjoy the rest of the day. Exercise is one of the best ways to prevent heart disease, and it is also one of the best ways to treat it once you have been diagnosed with the disease.

Exercise is the best means to strengthen your heart after a heart attack and restore you to a normal life. But the goal of this book is to catch you before you have that heart attack. The best medicine is prevention. So let's not waste any time.

Research has shown that regular exercise has a protective effect against dying from all causes, not just heart disease. Men who walked 3 miles 5 times a week had 75% less the risk of dying compared with couch potatoes their same age. There are sensationalized stories about athletes dying of a heart attack during exercise. It puts the fear in all of us and gives us one more excuse not to exercise. But the real truth is that out-of-shape men are over 100 times more likely to die of a heart attack during such simple things as running for the bus or shoveling snow than their exercising neighbors. Life has risks, but exercise does more to buffer you from the risk of heart attack and death than any pill.

BEFORE YOU BEGIN

I appreciate your caution in starting a program on your own. You're right to be cautious. There are risks when patients with heart disease exercise, but the risks of not exercising far outweigh the risks of activity. So you don't get to use this as an excuse for not starting. We'll discuss how to get started safely and the things to watch out for while you are exercising.

Before starting any exercise program, you should get clearance from your doctor. Sounds familiar, I know. But it is much more than a way for me to cover my legal behind. Depending on the severity of your disease, your physician may want you to have a stress test to evaluate your heart function before starting on your own. It is a very good idea. A resting ECG (electrocardiogram, which gives a picture of how your heart is functioning) only gives us a picture of your heart when it is at rest—not under stress. To exercise safely on your own, your doctor needs to see how your heart performs under the stress of exercise. This will unmask problems that aren't evident otherwise.

If you have been diagnosed with heart disease, have ongoing chest pain, or have worsening shortness of breath, then you must get clearance from your doctor before starting *any* exercise program. Chest pain and shortness of breath are warning signs that must never be ignored and should be evaluated whether or not you plan to start exercising. We know that regular exercise will help protect you from developing heart disease. But vigorous activity (more than 60% of your maximum) may actually cause a heart attack in a very few selected people. So go see your doctor before you begin a strenuous program to make sure you're not one of those unlucky ones.

In addition, if you are a man over the age of 45 or a woman over the age of 50, then it is strongly recommended that you have a stress test before starting a vigorous exercise program. These recommendations are from the American College of Sports Medicine based on the prevalence of heart disease in this country. Please check with your doctor. These recommendations are for first-time exercisers. For those of you who are symptom free, I encourage you to start your walking program while you're waiting for that doctor's appointment. Light activity is the perfect way to start and is not associated with increased cardiac risk. In fact, that is how I will tell you to start your program anyway.

SAFETY PRECAUTIONS

The following precautions are signals that your heart is not getting enough oxygen/blood flow, and that worries physicians because it may signal a progression of your disease. These signs should not be ignored. If you have followed my advice and had a thorough physical exam and stress test before you started your exercise program, then it is unlikely that these danger signs will occur:

1. Listen closely to your body for signs of overexertion. If you feel discomfort or pain in your chest, neck, arm, stomach, or back, then decrease your exercise intensity, cool down with very slow walking for 5 minutes, and contact your doctor before your next exercise session. This pain may be a signal that your heart is not getting enough oxygen. It is called ischemia and must be evaluated with some urgency. In addition to pain, you must also pay attention to unaccustomed shortness of breath. If you are getting short of breath much earlier in your workout or at an easier workload, then you need to slow down, stop, and notify your physician immediately.

2. If you feel dizzy or light-headed during your normal workout, then begin your cooldown with slow walking and notify your doctor as soon as possible.

3. If you feel nauseous during exercise, then you must view this as a warning sign, stop exercising with a 5-minute cooldown, and notify your doctor as soon as possible.

4. Be cautious about exercising in extreme humidity, heat, or cold temperatures. Both temperature extremes increase the workload on your heart and can put you at risk. Increased humidity makes it very difficult for your body to cool itself, which puts a tremendous stress on your heart. If you are unsure, then it is best to move your exercise indoors on those days where outdoor conditions could stress your heart. Stay well hydrated. Your thirst mechanism is not very sensitive, so you should actually drink water before you feel thirsty. Once you feel thirsty, you are already behind the eight ball.

5. If you are taking certain blood pressure medications, beta-blockers, and diuretics, then you also need to be especially careful about exercising in the heat. You are more susceptible to heat illness and to a drop in your blood sugar when you exercise in a hot and/or humid

environment. So if you are going to exercise in the heat, then you must know the warning signs of heat illness, wear clothing that helps wick away the sweat to keep you cool (no rubber pants, please), exercise during the cooler times of day, and adjust your exercise intensity downward when it is hot outside.

6. Cooldown is especially important if you are taking medication for your heart or to control your blood pressure. Alpha-blockers, calcium channel blockers, and vasodilators can cause an abrupt fall in your blood pressure if you stop exercising suddenly. To prevent a sudden drop in blood pressure (and the fainting that could result), you must gradually cool down by slowly walking for about 10 minutes after your exercise session. If you don't know what kind of blood pressure medication you are taking, then ask your doctor. It's your responsibility to know.

7. Remember that calcium channel blockers and beta-blockers (two medications used to treat heart disease and hypertension) will blunt your heart rate's response to exercise. You may be working very, very hard, but your heart rate is still in the lazy zone according to your heart rate monitor. For you, heart rate is not a good indicator of your exercise intensity. Leave the monitor at home. Instead, I recommend monitoring your breathing rate and how hard you feel you are working as your guide to your exercise intensity.

8. And lastly, the timing of your exercise program is important if you take heart or blood pressure medication. You don't want exercise to block absorption of your medications. With moderate- to high-intensity exercise, blood is shunted away from your stomach and directed to your working muscles. So wait 2–3 hours after taking your medication before you start to exercise vigorously. There should be no problem with a light walk right after you take your pills. The safe window is to exercise 3–10 hours after your take your medication. That way your medications will have their full protective effect during your exercise session.

LET'S GET STARTED: YOUR EXERCISE PROGRAM

We've discussed how exercise can treat your heart disease. It will strengthen your heart, your arteries, and your veins and even make your muscles more efficient at using oxygen. After beginning a regular exercise program, just getting through the day will be much easier since you are stronger and have more energy. Exercise can prevent heart attacks and buffer the severity of a heart attack if it occurs.

A well-rounded exercise program includes four components: aerobic exercise, strength training, balance, and flexibility. Regardless of your disease and fitness level, each of these should be part of your exercise routine. But because you have coronary artery disease, the focus of your exercise program will be on heart health and weight loss. To treat your heart disease and optimize your body weight, the focus of your exercise program needs to be on aerobic exercise. If your exercise time is limited, then put your time into aerobics or cardio as it is now called. Here is the outline of your exercise program:

Warm-up for 10 minutes before starting each exercise session.

Aerobic exercise for 10 minutes 3 days a week initially, then over the next 2 months, progress to 30 minutes 4–5 days a week. Start at an exercise intensity of 4–5 on the perceived exertion scale if you are new to exercise. Work up to an intensity that is 60%–70% of your max (6–7 on the perceived exertion scale) over the next 3 months.

Resistance training for 15–30 minutes 3 days a week to supplement your aerobic work. Do 15–20 reps of each exercise using lighter weights. And breathe with every movement to avoid dangerous increases in your blood pressure and stress on your heart.

Cooldown for 10–15 minutes after each session.

These are your guidelines. The most important thing you can do is learn to listen to your body and adapt how hard and how long you exercise to its needs. If your knees are hurting during exercise and continue to hurt for several hours after you're done, then that is a signal that you pushed too hard and need to slow down the next session. If you are no longer winded, then that is a signal that your body is getting stronger and you need to pick up your pace to continue to provide an exercise challenge. If you are exercising and just don't have the energy or the drive to continue, then listen to your body and stop for the day. Pat yourself on the back for the work that you have done and go home. You can work harder the next time. Remember, you don't have to be an aerobic animal every day to make significant progress. But you do need to listen to your body and respect what it is telling you. That is especially true if you have heart disease. On the flip side, if you can't find the motivation to get started, then just tell yourself to go for a 10-minute walk. Just get yourself off the couch and move. I'll bet once you get going, your walk time turns from 10 minutes to 30 minutes. But if it doesn't, then still pat yourself on the back for overcoming your inertia and taking a positive step for yourself.

WARM-UP (5-10 minutes before every exercise session)

Three hours after taking your heart medications, you will start with a slow walk and gradually increase your pace over the next 5–10 minutes until your body has slowly and carefully warmed up. Your goal is to increase your pace gradually until you are working at a 5/10 on the Borg scale (breathing heavy but you can still talk easily). At the end of your warm-up phase, your body literally feels warm and you are breathing heavily. Now you are ready to begin your aerobic work. Your warm-up and cooldown are especially important to ease your heart into and out of the demands of exercise. Don't skip this step.

AEROBIC EXERCISE (10–30 minutes 3–5 days a week)

How hard should you exercise, and what intensity is safe if you have heart disease? Obviously, the safe exercise intensity varies with the extent of your heart disease. Your doctor can give you your specific guidelines. Anyone who is sedentary and beginning an exercise program for the first time should start at a very low intensity (40%–50% maximum or a perceived exertion of 4–5) and gradually increase your effort as tolerated. Start with just 10–15 minutes of exercise a day. Do this 3–4 times a week. The most important thing you can do is find what you enjoy. Walking, biking, hiking, rowing, dancing are all very good aerobic activities. Even gardening and vacuuming are aerobic if you increase your heart rate and are breathing heavy for 30 minutes.

If you have been exercising on a regular basis and are using this book to get smarter and more efficient about what you do, then start with 30 minutes of aerobic work. Your goal is eventually 30–40 minutes per day at an exertion level of 5–7 on the perceived exertion scale. Make your exercise session a scheduled part of your workweek, and put it on your calendar just like you do all your important appointments. And if excess body fat is adding or contributing to your heart disease, elevated blood pressure, and high cholesterol (and I promise you that it is), then exercising 5 days a week for 40 minutes is definitely indicated to help burn off that stored fat. It took you time to put that fat on, and it will take a time commitment to burn it off.

RESISTANCE EXERCISES (15–30 minutes 3 days a week)

I have limited the number of resistance exercises included in this chapter, because weight training should not be the primary focus of your exercise routine. Spend the majority of your time doing aerobic exercise. If you have other problems like low back pain or arthritis, then please read that chapter and adjust your weight training according the recommendations in that chapter. The exercises I have selected here are for people with no painful physical limitations. These exercises are designed to use a number of muscle groups at a time to optimize the efficiency of your weight training session so you have more time for cardio work. Select one or two exercises from each group to provide a complete full-body workout. You should use a weight that allows you to easily do 15–20 reps without straining. So pick a weight that you can lift with perfect form 15 times. But make sure it's heavy enough that you are working hard by repetition number 20. Do the full-body workout 3 days a week. Additional exercises are given so you can change your routine every 4–6 weeks.

Once you are a pro and can do all these exercises safely and with perfect form, I want you to take them onto a balance board like a BOSU board. This will add a new dimension of difficulty and stress and strengthen your muscles even more.

A second way to up your intensity is to add a pause during the exercise. For example, pause halfway down during your push-up hold for 2 seconds and then continue the movement. The way to continue to improve is by making changes in your exercise program that continue to stress your muscles. Stay out of your comfort zone and find ways to mix up your exercise routine.

LEGS

Pick one exercise from each of the leg sections: glutes, hamstrings, and calves. The exercises in these sections have good overlap, so you'll be working the same muscles several ways, just with a different focus in each grouping. Start with just one exercise per group and later increase the number to continue to challenge your muscles. Pick a new exercise every 4–6 weeks. And don't forget the balance exercises at the end of this section.

LEGS–QUADS

Sit to Stand

You will be surprised how difficult this really is.

Sit on a firm straight-backed chair. Engage your core (tighten your stomach like someone was going to punch you in the gut). With stomach strong, slowly stand up. Use your legs, not your arms, to lift your body off the chair. If you cannot stand without using your arms, then allow them to assist you—but no more than necessary. Slowly lower back to the seated position, but halfway down, pause for a count of 2 or 4, then continue to the seated position. Do as many as you can with perfect form (targets quadriceps, core).

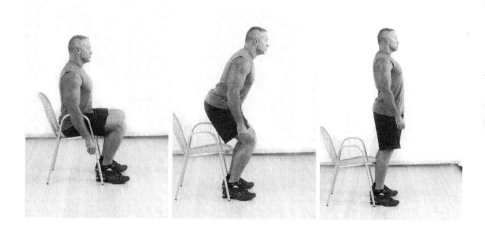

Step Up

Stand straight with your stomach strong. Step your right foot onto first step and slowly straighten leg. Keep toes facing front. Bring left foot up to touch step by right ankle, then slowly lower your weight to count of 4 onto left leg. Don't push off back leg. Move slowly so the muscles, and not the momentum, do the work. As you stand up, press your weight through the heel, not the ball, of your foot. Repeat 12–15 times with each leg. When the stair step becomes easy, carry 5–10 lb. dumbbells to increase difficulty; just keep breathing (targets quadriceps and glutes, balance).

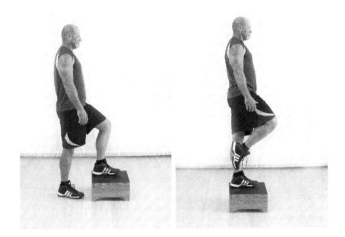

Wall Squat

Stand with a fitness ball between you and a wall. Rest your lower back against the fitness ball. Your feet should be shoulder width apart and about 3 feet away from the wall. Slowly bend your knees till your thighs are parallel to the floor or as low as you can go. Make sure you keep your knees directly over your toes. Pause and then squeeze your buttocks as you return to the standing position. Work up to 15-20 reps. As this gets easier deepen your knee bend to optimize quadriceps strengthening. But keep breathing (targets quadriceps, glutes).

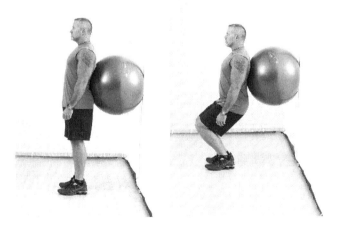

Dumbbell Split Squat

Step your right foot forward about 12 inches and your left leg back about 12 inches. Keep your chest up and stomach tight, bend both knees, and lower your body to a slow count of 4 and then straighten your legs to the same slow count. Stop when your form begins to slip. Do 15–20 reps. For added difficulty, hold your arms over your head or hold 5–10 lb. dumbbells at your sides (targets quadriceps, hamstrings, and glutes, balance).

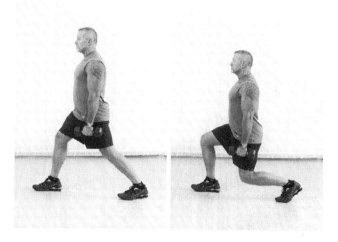

Lying Leg Lifts in 3 Positions

Lie on your right side with your head supported on your right arm. Keep both legs straight with your toes pointed forward. Slowly lift your left leg, keeping your knee straight and your toes pointing forward. You will feel the muscles of your outer thigh engage. Raise your leg to the count of 2, pause, and then lower to the count of 2. Repeat 8 times.

Now do the same exercise with your toes and knee pointing at the ceiling. As your raise your leg, you will feel your thigh muscles doing the work. Raise your leg to the count of 2, pause, and then lower to the count of 2. Lastly, turn your leg so your toes and knee point to the floor. You will have to let your hip drop forward. Keep your knee facing the floor as you lift your leg to the count of 2 and lower to the count of 2. You will feel the muscles in the back of your leg engage to do the work of lifting your leg. Repeat 8 times. Roll on your other side and repeat the whole exercise with your left leg (targets quadriceps, hamstrings, leg abductors).

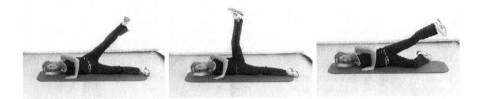

LEGS–HAMSTRINGS

Pick one of these exercises to start with. Change every 4–6 weeks.

Hip Bridge

Lying on your back with heels tucked close to your buttocks, lift your buttocks off the ground so your body forms a straight line from knees to shoulders. Hold for 2 seconds, then slowly lower over a 2-second count. Do 15–20 reps (targets hamstrings, glutes, and low back).

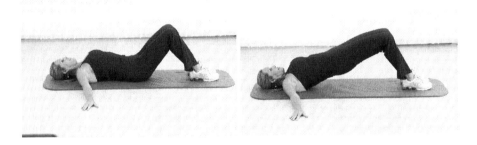

For added difficulty, straighten your right leg from the knee and do the movement using only the left leg to lift your body. Keep the right leg straight during the exercise. Do 8–12 reps on each side.

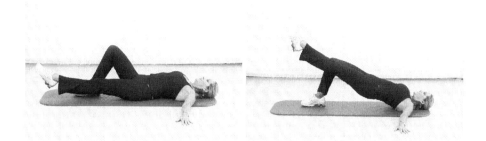

For even more difficulty, straighten your right leg with your toes pointing at the ceiling. Keep your leg pointed toward the ceiling as you raise your body with your left leg. Do 8–12 reps, then repeat with the left leg straight.

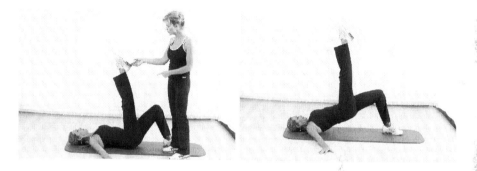

Hamstring Ball Roll

Lie on your back with your legs straight and your calves resting on a stability ball. You are in a straight line from your shoulders to your heels. Bend your knees and roll the ball toward your buttocks. Keep your hips elevated, and you will feel your hamstrings and buttocks working as you bring the stability ball as close to your buttocks as you can. Just your heels should be resting on the ball at this time. It is easiest to do this exercise with your arms extended out to the side on the floor for balance. Do 15–20 repetitions. For added difficulty and better core strengthening, keep your arms at your sides (targets hamstrings, low back, and glutes).

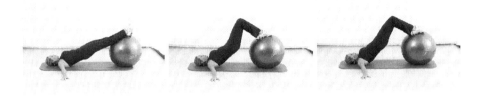

Fire Hydrant

Kneel on all fours on a mat and place a 1 or 3 lb. weight behind your right knee. Squeeze your leg muscles so that the dumbbell stays locked in place. Keeping your back flat and your head down, slowly raise your right leg until your thigh is parallel with the floor. Pause and then lower your right leg to the starting position. Do 15–20 reps with each leg (targets hamstrings and glutes).

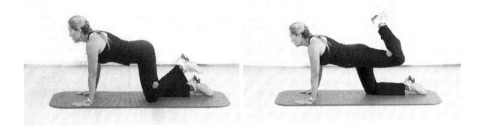

LEGS–CALVES

Pick one of these exercises to start with. Change every 4–6 weeks. And remember that many of the balance exercises strengthen your calves as well.

Seated Calf Raise

Sit with 5 or 10 lb. dumbbells resting on each knee. Slowly lift your knees and come up on the balls of your feet. Pause for a count of 2 and then slowly lower. Make sure that you're using your calves to raise the weights and not your arms. Repeat 15–20 times (targets calves).

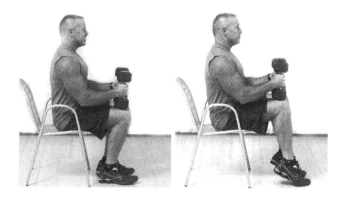

Standing Calf Raise

Stand on a step or a block with the toes and ball of your right foot at the edge of the step. Hold on to a wall or chair with your left hand for balance. Cross your left foot behind your right ankle and balance yourself on the ball of your right foot. Lower your heel as far as you can till you feel a stretch in the back of your calf. Lift your heel as high as you can, pause, and return to the starting position. Do 10–15 reps and repeat with the left leg (targets calves, balance).

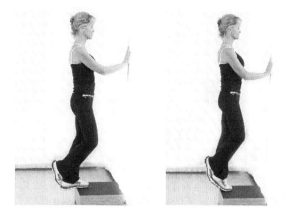

BALANCE

Change exercises every 4–6 weeks or take any of the exercises you do standing on 2 feet and try them on one foot.

Marching in Place

Stand tall with your core strong (say *sshhh* to engage your abdominal muscles). March in place slowly, lifting your knees as high as you can. When this is easy, do it on a folded towel or soft cushion.

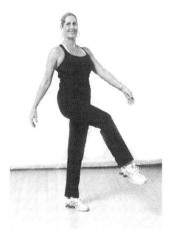

Eyes Closed

Stand on a thick folded towel with your feet shoulder width apart. Stand tall with your abdominal muscles engaged (say *sshhh* to engage them). Close your eyes and visualize the upright position.

Balance on One Leg

Stand with your hand on a chair or bar for support. Shift your weight to your left leg and lift the right leg off the floor. Try letting go of your support or only resting your fingertips on the bar for balance. Your goal is to stand on one leg for 30 seconds. Turn around and repeat it standing on your right leg.

Advanced

Fold a bath towel several times over, place it on the floor, and stand on the center of the towel. This will give you a slightly unstable surface because the towel is soft.

Advanced

Try doing the one-leg balance with your eyes shut. Keep the chair back close so you can steady yourself as needed.

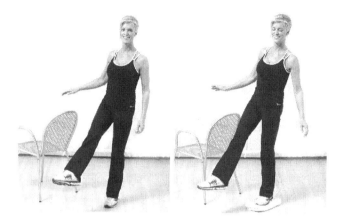

Toe-Stand Balance

Stand facing a sturdy chair or bar with your hands resting lightly on it. Rise up onto your toes and try to let go of the chair and balance for a count of 10. When you are an expert, raise up on your toes and, still holding on gently, shift your weight to the right leg and try to balance on your toes on one leg. You will feel the muscles of your entire leg and your core engage. Keep your head high and stomach strong (say *sshhh*).

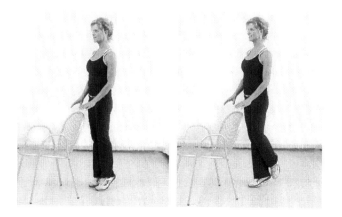

Step-ups on a Stair

Stand straight with stomach strong, holding on to handrail. Step your right foot onto first step and slowly straighten leg. Keep toes facing front. Bring left foot up to touch step by right ankle, then slowly lower your weight to count of 4 onto left leg. Repeat 10 times with each leg. Don't push off back leg. Move slowly so the muscles, and not the momentum, do the work. As you stand up, press your weight through the heel, not the ball, of your foot.

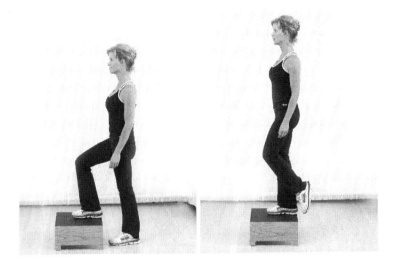

Lunge with Trunk Rotation

Stand with your right leg one stride in front of the left with the left heel lifted, abdominals tensed, and your arms out at your side at shoulder height. Bend both knees and lower your hips directly between the two legs so your right thigh is parallel with the floor. Make sure your knees are in line with your toes. Use your hip and thigh muscles to bring your left leg through and forward till the left knee is at hip level. As your raise your left leg, twist your body so you look over your left thigh. Return to the starting position and repeat 8 times. Then alternate legs and repeat with the right leg (targets quadriceps, hamstrings, glutes, calves, abdominals, and lower back).

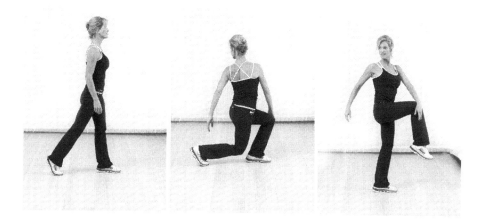

CORE

Although you'll see everyone in the gym dropping to do 50 sit-ups, they are defeating the purpose on several fronts. The first problem is the number 50. Any exercise you do where you can do more than 20 is not building strength efficiently. Your best bet is to slow down the exercise so you recruit more muscle fibers and build strength efficiently. Doing 50 sit-ups does not provide enough muscle resistance to build strength. Working your abs slowly or adding weight will recruit the maximal number of muscle fibers and provide optimal strength gains. Find 1 or 2 exercises that are hard enough that you can only do 15–20 reps.

The second problem is with the word *sit-up*. It's a bad choice of an exercise to build core strength. You see, any exercise where you raise your body up from the floor is using your hip flexor muscles far more than it uses your abdominal muscles. So with the classic sit-up, you are training your hip flexors but not your abdominal/core muscles. The sit-up is not only ineffective, but it is also potentially dangerous. It can easily strain your low back, a situation we want to avoid. The exercises that follow are safe for your back and will develop all four of your abdominal muscles, providing the strong core you need. Your core muscles include your rectus abdominis muscle, which is your six-pack. But there are three other sets of muscles that run underneath the rectus muscles. These three sets of muscles run diagonally and across your belly and are the ones we want to strengthen. The following exercises focus on strengthening these. Core also includes your low back muscles. They work in tandem with your abdominal muscles to provide support for your back. Pick a combination of exercises that work both. You should do 2–3 of the following exercises as part of your weight training program. After 4–6 weeks, switch exercises.

Half Locust

Lie on your belly, chin on the floor, arms stretched back alongside your body with palms down. With your toes pointed, lift your right leg a few inches off the floor. Hold for several seconds, then slowly lower. Do 15–20 reps; switch legs and repeat (targets back).

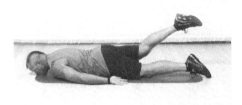

Medicine Ball Twist

Sit on the floor with your legs extended and your back straight. Place a medicine ball (start with a light ball) next to your right hip. Twist and pick up the ball and place it beside the opposite hip. Repeat on each side for a total of 12–15 reps.

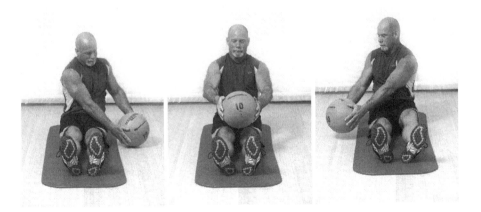

Resistance One-Leg Crunch

Lie on your back with your knees bent with your feet on the floor. Lift your right knee and resist the movement with your right arm. Hold for a count of 2 and then return to the starting position. Repeat on the left. That is 1 repetition. Work up so you can do 8–12 reps (targets abs).

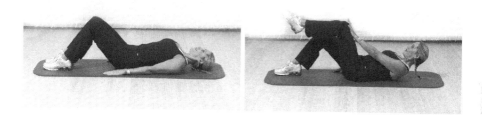

Superman

This works your back extensor muscles with minimal stress on your spine compared to more traditional back exercises. Kneel on your hands and knees. Keep your stomach tight (like you're being punched), but keep the normal arch in your lower back. Straighten your right leg behind you, keeping it at hip level. Then raise your right arm so it extends straight out at ear level. Keep both your outstretched arm and leg parallel to the floor. Hold for a count of 4, then repeat on the other side. Do 12–15 repetitions each side (targets lower back, glutes, and hamstrings).

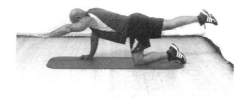

When that becomes simple, start from a standard push-up position and raise your left leg while maintaining the perfect push-up position (targets abdominals, back, hamstrings, and glutes).

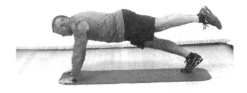

Pelvic Tilt

On the floor, lie on your back with your knees bent. Your feet are flat on the floor and your arms at your sides, palms facing the ground. To a count of 2, slowly roll your pelvis so that hips and lower back are off the floor while upper back and shoulders remain in place. Hold for a count of 2, then slowly lower. Repeat 12–15 times (targets back, glutes, and abs).

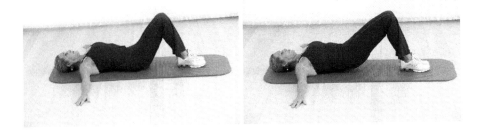

One-Leg Abdominal Crunch

Lie on your back with a small rolled-up towel under your lower back. Bring your knees to your chest. Hold your legs close together with your knees above your hips. Raise both arms straight above your shoulders. Engage your stomach (like you're being punched). While keeping your abdominal muscles tight, slowly lower your right foot as low as you can without letting your back lift off the floor. Bring your leg back to the starting position and repeat with the left leg. Repeat 8 times, alternating legs. If you start to feel a strain in your back, then limit the range of motion of your legs and focus on keeping your stomach strong (targets abdominals, hip flexors).

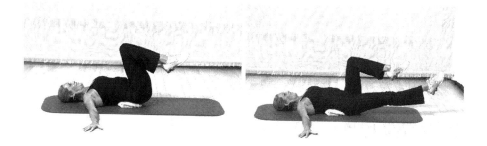

Bicycle

Lie on your back and lift your legs straight in the air. Keep your hands on your stomach to make sure it stays strong and your back stays flat on the floor. Move your legs like you are pedaling a bike. Do this for 30 seconds (targets abs).

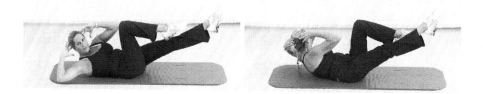

Plank

This is one of my favorite core-strengthening exercises.

Assume a modified push-up position with your forearms resting on the floor. Elbows should be under your shoulders and bent at 90 degrees. Keep your torso steady and your body in a straight line from your head to your toes. Do not let your stomach sag. Hold for as long as you can. Your goal is to hold this for 30 seconds (targets core-stabilizing muscles).

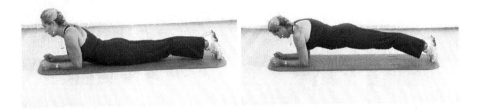

Bench Twist

Lie facedown on an exercise bench or your bed with your torso hanging off the end. Raise your torso until you are in a straight line and hold for a count of 4. Slowly lower your torso so it is hanging off the end of the bench again. Repeat 8–10 times (targets back).

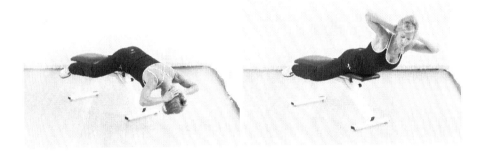

Advanced

After you raise your torso, extend your arms out to the side so you are in a school-yard airplane position. Gently rotate your torso so your head and shoulders are facing the wall to your right. Return to the starting position and then repeat on the left. Do 8–10 repetitions.

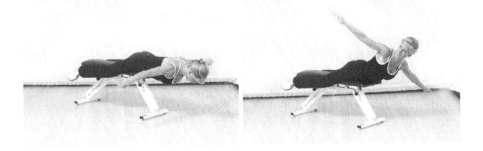

UPPER BACK

This section supplements the lower back work found in the core section with upper back work. This should be one of your target spots as we fight the shoulders slump of old age. You can combat the humped posture with a strong back and a balance between chest and upper back strength. In other words, don't overdo your chest work just because it is an area you can see and admire. What your admirers really love is good posture and squared-off shoulders. Pick one to two exercises from this section and select a new exercise every 4–6 weeks

Dumbbell Single-Arm Row

Holding a dumbbell in your right hand, place your left knee and left hand on a bench. Your right arm should be straight and hang just in front of your shoulder. Keeping your back flat and right elbow close to your body, pull the dumbbell up and back toward your hip. Pause and then slowly lower the weight. Repeat 15–20 times, then switch sides (targets upper back).

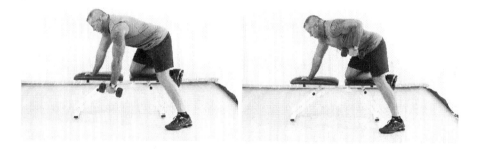

Dumbbell Row with Rotation

Stand with your feet shoulder width apart and hold a 1 or 3 lb. dumbbell in each hand. Bend forward at the waist. Keep your back flat and your core strong. Bend your knees and let the dumbbells hang in front of your thighs, palms facing each other. Start by pulling your right arm up to your rib cage while rotating your shoulders and torso as far as you can to the right. Pause and then slowly lower your right arm while pulling your left arm up to your chest and rotating your body to the left. Remember to keep your core rock-hard strong during the entire exercise. Do 15–20 reps each side (targets upper back and core).

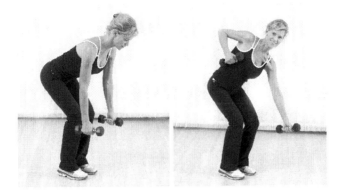

Wall Slide

Stand with your buttocks, upper back and head against the wall. Raise your arms over your head so your shoulders, elbows, and wrists also touch the wall. Maintaining these points of contact, bend your arms until your elbows are tucked in at your sides. You should feel a contraction in your shoulders and the muscles between your shoulder blades. Reverse the move. Do 10 repetitions (targets upper back).

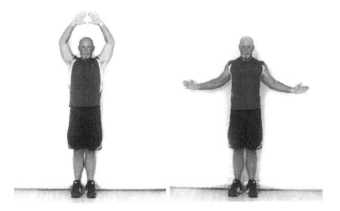

Lat Pull Down

Sit at the lat pull-down station. Adjust the leg pads so your legs fit secure underneath. Grab the bar and begin by pulling your shoulder blades down and together. Keep them pinched tight and then pull the bar down toward the floor (or if you are using a bar, then pull it down to chest height). Keep your back straight and move slowly through the full range of motion. Do 15–20 reps (targets back).

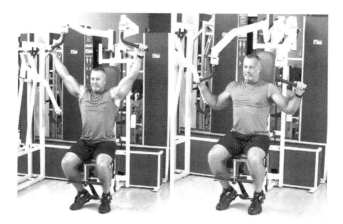

SHOULDERS

Select one or two exercises from this section and change exercises every 4–6 weeks.

Forward and Lateral Shoulder Raise

Stand holding a 1–3 lb. dumbbell in each hand. With arms straight, lift your right arm in front of your body to shoulder level. At the same time, lift your left arm straight out to the side, stopping when it is shoulder height also. Pause for a 1–2 count and then slowly lower. Then lift the left arm to the front and your right arm to the side. Do not lift your arms beyond shoulder level. Pause and then slowly lower. Repeat 15–20 times (targets shoulders and abs).

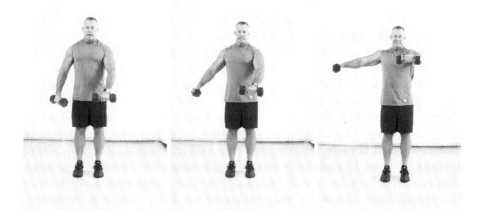

Dumbbell Upright Row

Stand holding a pair of dumbbells in front of your thighs, arms straight and palms facing your body. Lift your upper arms and bring the dumbbells up until your hands are just below your chin. Pause and then lower the weight back to the starting position. Do 15–20 reps (targets shoulders).

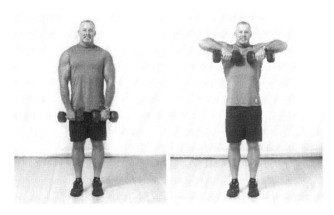

Internal/External Rotation

This is a great one to stabilize your shoulder girdle and prevent injuries.

Stand with your arm at your side, a 1–3 lb. dumbbell in your hand. Bend your elbow at 90 degrees so your forearm and hand point forward with your palm facing toward your body. Slowly bring your arm across your body until your hand touches your abdomen. Return to the starting position. Keep your elbow in a fixed position so your shoulder rotator cuff muscles do all the work. Then repeat the exercise so that your hands rotate away from your body and face out in either direction. Again, keep your elbows at a 90-degree angle and fixed in position. Do 15–20 reps (targets shoulders, internal and external rotators).

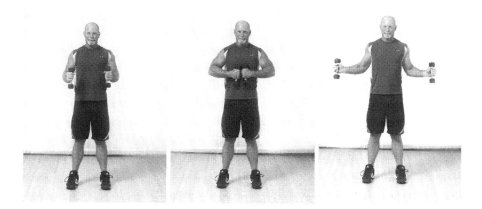

Alternating Shoulder Dumbbell Press

By alternating your arms, you also get core strengthening with the exercise.

Sit with your back supported. Engage your core (like you are preparing to be punched). This will provide a solid core to protect your back and double the value of the exercise by working your stomach muscles. Hold a 1–3 lb. dumbbell in each hand at shoulder level with palms facing each other. Press the dumbbell in your right hand straight above you until your arm is straight and the weight is above your head. Then slowly lower the weight to the starting position. Repeat on the left. Do a total of 15–20 per side (targets shoulders and core).

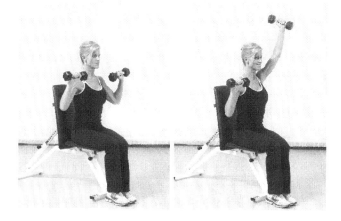

Advanced

Do the same exercise standing or stand on one leg to challenge your core. Keep your abdominal muscles engaged.

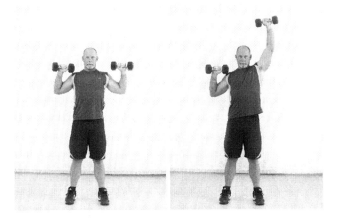

Lateral Raises 3 Ways

This is one of my favorite exercises and part of my exercise routine. To use all three heads of the deltoid, you will do the standard lateral raise using three different hand positions. Do this exercise with low weight and slow, controlled movements.

Stand tall, stomach firm, holding a 1, 3, or 5 lb. dumbbell in each hand. With your hands facing forward and arms straight, slowly raise both dumbbells at a 45-degree angle to shoulder level. Your thumbs should be pointing at the ceiling. Do not raise them above shoulder level. Slowly lower to the count of 2 or 4. You will feel this primarily in the anterior head of the deltoid (your shoulder muscle).

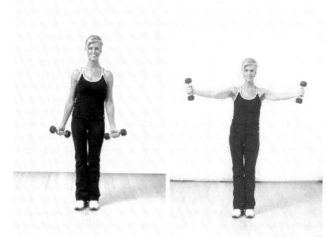

Next, turn your hands to face each other and lift the dumbbells slowly to the side. All your knuckles will be directed toward the ceiling. Do not raise them above shoulder level. This will strengthen the middle head of the deltoid. Slowly lower.

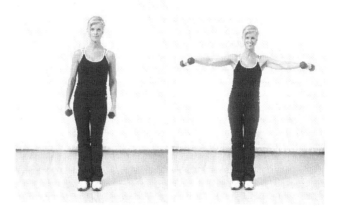

Lastly, turn your hands facing the back with your pinkies on top. Slowly lift to the side, again stopping at shoulder height. You will feel this engage the posterior head of the deltoid. Slowly lower. Repeat the entire set (all three moves are 1 set) 12 times.

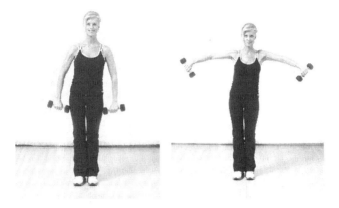

CHEST

Select one exercise from this section and pick new exercises to try every 4–6 weeks.

Wall Push-ups (the perfect beginner's exercise)

Stand at arm's length from the wall. Put both hands on the wall at chest level. Slowly bend your elbows to the count of 4 and then slowly straighten them. Repeat 12 times. When this is easy, go to the modified push-up below (targets chest).

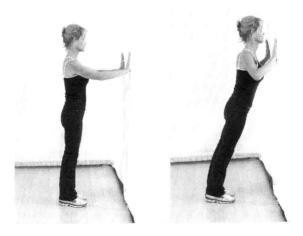

Push-ups on Knees

I know these are girl push-ups, but done correctly, they will result in impressive improvements in your strength. Once you can do 12 of these with perfect form, then it is time to do them in the regular push-up position. Keep your core strong throughout the push-up by maintaining a straight line from your knees to the top of your head.

Kneel on the floor with your knees on a pad. Walk your arms out until your body is in a straight line with your knees bent. In this modified push-up position, I want you to slowly lower your body (keeping a straight line from the tip of your head to your knees) until you are barely touching the floor and then slowly return to the starting position, keeping perfect form (targets chest).

Do 6–12 reps in each of the three-hand positions illustrated.

A) Normal push-up position—elbows are at a 90-degree angle with your hands right under your elbows.

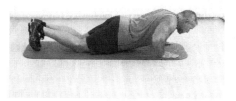

B) Wide-arm position—hands are placed out past your elbows so the angle of your elbows is about 120 degrees.

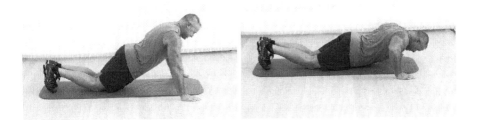

C) Diamond—place your hands so that your thumb and index fingers touch each other and make the shape of a diamond.

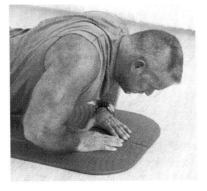

Dumbbell Incline Bench Press

Lie faceup on an incline bench and hold 3–5 lb. dumbbells along the outside of your chest with elbows bent and palms facing inward. Slowly press the weight straight above your chest (see picture). Pause and then slowly lower. Do 15–20 reps (targets chest).

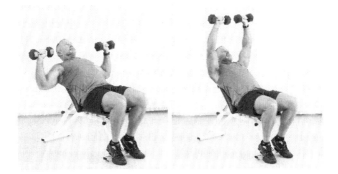

Dumbbell Incline Fly

Lie faceup on an incline bench. Hold 3–5 lb. dumbbells straight over your chest with your palms facing each other. Slowly open your arms, keeping your hands in line with your shoulders. Stop when the weights are level with your chest. Pause and return to the starting position. Repeat 15–20 times (targets chest).

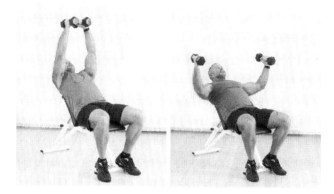

COOLDOWN (10-15 minutes after every exercise session)

The cooldown is important to minimize muscle soreness and fatigue. During exercise, your body accumulates lactic acid (a by-product of muscle work). We associate lactic acid buildup with muscle soreness. The cooldown period gives your body a chance to clear the lactic acid from your muscles, so it minimizes postworkout discomfort.

Do not stop exercising abruptly. If you simply stop after exercising vigorously, then there is a good chance your blood pressure will drop and you will get light-headed and dizzy. Keep moving. It's what all the experts say and for very good reason. Especially if you have any history of coronary artery disease, you need to make the cooldown period an important priority. Think of the cooldown period as "active rest," where you are gently returning your body to its pre-exercise state. Walk slowly for about 10 minutes after you finish exercising to gently return your heart rate to its resting level. Or you can simply do a slower version of whatever exercise you were doing. Continue walking until you are breathing normally and can easily carry on a conversation. Your cooldown period is the best time to stretch. But wait until your heart rate has slowed and is approaching your resting value. If you suffer from arthritis, then this is the perfect time to focus on those painful joints with gentle stretches to maintain their range of motion and minimize their pain. Refer to the arthritis chapter for stretches specific for your joint pain.

And don't forget to rehydrate. Unless you have been exercising at a high intensity for an hour or more, water is the best fluid for rehydration. None of us need the calories of the electrolyte drinks, and rarely do we lose enough salt with routine exercise to require extra salt found in these sport drinks.

GENERAL STRETCHES FOR YOUR COOLDOWN

Maintaining flexibility of your muscles will increase your range of motion and keep you agile and prevent injuries. The most important way to increase your flexibility is to do every resistance exercise through the full range of movement. Exercises like lunges, squats, and even push-ups should be done by moving your body through its full *pain-free* range of motion. As you move your body as far as it can, make sure you keep good form during every repetition.

But because they feel so good, I have included my favorite stretches. When you do these stretches, start slowly, breathe deeply, and push just to the limit of pain. You will find that as your joint warms up, you will be able to go a little farther each time. Use your breath to help you relax into each stretch. Take a slow, deep breath in through your nose and then relax into the stretch as you exhale through your mouth. Think about your breath and consciously breathe deep in through your nose, filling your lungs down to their bases. This will help you relax and make the most of each stretch. Bouncing or forcing the stretch is actually counterproductive. *Do not bounce.* Plan to do the majority of your stretching program while you are cooling down—while your muscles are still warm from exercising.

Kneeling Quad Stretch

Kneel with your right leg bent in front of you with your knee at a 90-degree angle and your left knee on a mat for cushioning. Keep your body vertical and gently press your hips forward to feel a stretch in the front of the left thigh and hip. Hold for a count of 10, then relax. Repeat 5–10 times and then repeat on the other side.

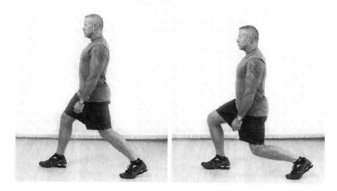

Quadriceps Standing Stretch

Stand facing a chair, holding on to the back lightly for balance. Bend the right knee and grab your ankle with your right hand. Hold for a count of 5, exhaling during the stretch. Try to balance by lifting your hands off the back of the chair on during the stretch to engage core strengthening.

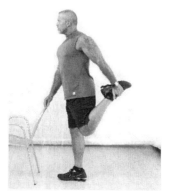

Piriformis Stretch

Lying on your back, bend your right knee with your knee at a 90-degree angle and your foot on the floor. Rest your left ankle on your right leg and let your knee relax out to the side. Gently pull your right knee to your chest and feel the stretch in the left buttock. Hold for a count of 5, exhaling during the stretch.

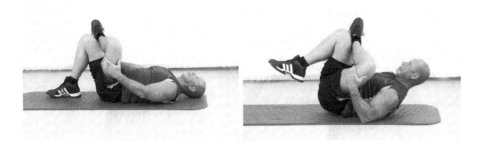

Lying Hamstring Stretch

Lie on your back with both legs straight on the floor and arms by your sides. Bring your right knee to your chest. Place both hands behind your right knee and slowly straighten your right leg. It is OK if you need to lower your right leg to get your knee straight. Hold the straight-leg position for a count of 5, slowly exhaling while you straighten it. Bend the knee again and repeat the exercise 5–10 times on each side.

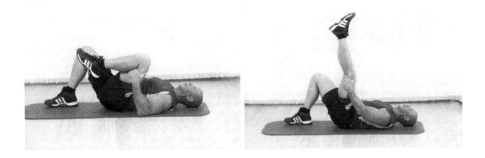

Calf Stretch

Stand on a bottom stair, holding on to the railing for support. Edge your feet back so your heels are off the step. Slowly rise up on your toes and hold for a count of 2. Then lower your body, keeping your knees straight until your heels are below the step and you feel a stretch up the back of your leg.

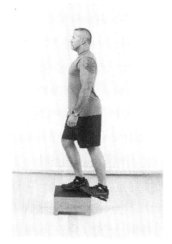

Floor Chest Stretch

Lie faceup on a foam roll with your head supported. Extend your arms out to your sides with your palms facing the ceiling. You will feel a stretch across your chest. Take slow, easy breaths and hold the stretch for 30 seconds. Repeat 3 times.

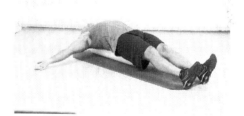

Supine Tuck and Curl

Lie flat on your back, knees bent and feet on the floor. Moving slowly, tilt your pelvis and lift your hips off the floor slightly, then lower. Do 6 reps.

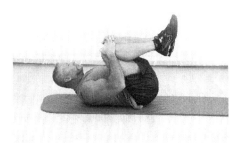

Knee-to-Chest Pose

Lie on your back with your legs fully extended. Draw one knee to your chest and hold it with both hands. Breathe in, and as you breathe out, pull your knee to your chest. Hold for 3–5 breaths. Switch legs and repeat.

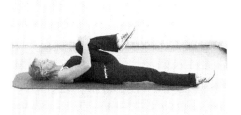

Trunk Twister

Lie on your back on the floor with your arms extended out at shoulder level. Raise your right leg until your toes point to the ceiling. Keeping your leg straight and your shoulders glued to the floor, slowly lower your leg across your body until your toe touches the floor on the left side of your body. Pause at the point that your shoulder wants to lift off the floor. Raise your leg back up in the air and then lower it to the floor. Repeat with your left leg. Do 5–10 repetitions on each side.

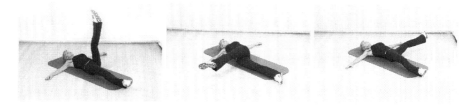

Side Stretch

Stand with your feet apart and stretch your arms over your head as you inhale. Draw a big circle with the fingertips of your right hand as you exhale through your mouth and reach to the side. Hold for a count of 2 and as you inhale and return to the upright position. Exhale and lower your arms to your sides. Repeat for a total of 8 on each side. This is a very relaxing way to finish your exercise session.

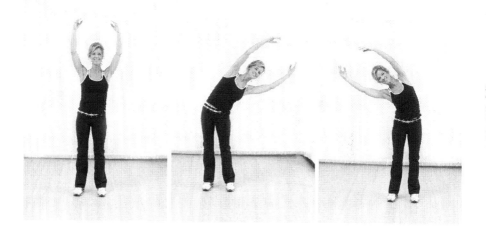

I believe the wise men who say that we are masters of our own fate. Our life is ours, our health is ours, our happiness is ours. Once you take responsibility for your health, you have the power to change it. Stop blaming, stop complaining, and slowly, with love and tenderness, pick yourself up off the couch and go for your first walk. It is the walk of your lifetime.

EXERCISE TO TREAT ARTHRITIS

Your lifestyle choices will determine whether you grow old debilitated by arthritis or not. You see, arthritis is another disease for which modern medicine has no cure. But with a combination of medications, exercise, and proper nutrition, you stand a pretty good chance of living a full, active, and pain-free life. Exercise has been shown in many studies to make a real difference in easing pain and returning function to people suffering from arthritis. It can also prevent the development of joint pain by keeping the muscles supporting each joint in top condition. The stronger the muscles, the more work they can do and the less wear and tear on your hips, knees, and even shoulders.

There are more than 100 different types of arthritis, but osteoarthritis is the most common and the most amenable to exercise intervention; that will be our focus. Osteoarthritis affects more than 27 million people. We think of osteoarthritis (also known as degenerative joint disease) as being a disease of old age, but joint pain is not an inevitable part of growing old. You see, if you took an x-ray of every person's hips and knees over the age of 40, almost 90% of them show evidence of joint degeneration. Yet these changes are asymptomatic (no pain). So just because it's there doesn't mean it hurts. Doctors only treat arthritis that is painful—if you don't hurt, then we don't care what the x-ray shows. Now, with the right diet and exercise program, you can prevent the arthritis seen on your x-rays from ever becoming painful. An anti-inflammatory diet is especially important for you—arthritis means inflammation of the joint. While the diet and exercise won't cure your disease, they will definitely help.

The most common joints to be affected are the weight-bearing joints—hips, knees, and feet. But it can affect any joint in the body including the ones in your spine. Although we can't predict who will get painful arthritis, there are certain risk factors that predispose you to developing the joint wear and tear that defines this disease. Some of these risk factors include obesity (a biggie), increasing age, a history of joint trauma, and your occupation (jobs that cause repetitive trauma and, overuse, can predispose you to developing arthritis).

WHY EXERCISE?

Osteoarthritis (I'll just call it *arthritis* for the rest of the chapter) results from wear and tear on the cartilage in the joint. The cartilage breaks down, and because of the increased stress on the bone (it has lost its cartilage cushion), new bone forms at the joint surface and along the bone margins called bone spurs. Exercise can't prevent you from developing arthritis, but by keeping the muscles that support your painful joints strong and flexible, you can minimize joint pain and disability. So you must exercise and maintain your ideal weight to keep your joints from hurting. You especially need to get exercising once those joints start to hurt to keep your arthritis pain from worsening. Yes, I said, when it hurts to move it, you should move it more. It's counterintuitive, I know.

When your knee hurts every time you walk, the natural reaction is to stop walking, alter your gait so it doesn't hurt, and spend much more time sitting. But that's the problem; that's how arthritis pain flares out of control. Inactivity weakens the muscles supporting the joint and stiffens the joint itself. Inactivity makes the disease much worse. This is the vicious cycle of arthritic pain. The one thing you need to do to combat the disease is to get moving, but when it hurts, this is very difficult. You see, this pain is like any other type of chronic pain—it feeds on inactivity. And not only does inactivity worsen your joint pain, but it can also lead to an increased risk of other conditions such as heart disease, hypertension, diabetes, depression, and obesity. You have to get moving.

Although arthritis is a disease of the elderly, you can't use your age as an excuse not to move. Regardless of how old you are (be it age 50 or 90), your body will see the benefits of a regular exercise program. Doctors know that you are never too old to start; you will benefit from exercise even if you start at age 90. But we also know you need to exercise the correct and safe way. Exercise programs that are prescribed incorrectly or performed incorrectly will flare your arthritis and make the disease worse. I have given you only the basics in the exercises that follow. After your doctor has cleared you medically to start your exercise program, ask them to write a prescription for physical therapy. A good therapist (and your success is very dependent on the quality of the therapist you work with) will teach you strengthening and stretching exercises that you can do at home. That exercise program must become part of your daily routine. With it, you can control your symptoms and keep your pain in check for the rest of your life. The exercises that follow are those used by physical therapists and exercise physiologists to treat arthritic pain. But the value of exercising with a therapist is manyfold; they will watch your exercise form and ensure you are getting the maximum benefit from each exercise and that you are doing them properly to avoid further injury. A good physical therapist will also customize your exercise program to your specific needs and limitations. If you don't have a physical therapist, then do your exercises with a friend who can watch how you perform each exercise and make sure your form is correct.

BEFORE YOU BEGIN

Before starting any exercise program, you should get clearance from your doctor. Sounds familiar, I know. But it is much more than a way for me to cover my legal behind. Patients with arthritis often have underlying heart disease and hypertension. There are risks when patients with high blood pressure and heart disease exercise, but the risks of *not* exercising far outweigh the risks of activity. So you don't get to use this as an excuse for not starting. I discuss how to get started safely and the things to watch out for while you are exercising in the chapters devoted to these diseases. And if you are a man over the age of 45 or a woman over the age of 50, then it is strongly recommended that you have a stress test before starting an exercise program. These recommendations are from the American College of Sports Medicine based on the prevalence of heart disease in this country. Please check with your doctor. These recommendations are for first-time exercisers. While you're waiting for that doctor's appointment, I encourage you to start your walking program. Light activity is the perfect way to start and is not associated with increased cardiac risk. In fact, that is how I will tell you to start your program anyway.

If you haven't been exercising for a while, then you may notice some increased pain and swelling of your joints after your exercise session. If your pain persists for longer than an hour after exercise and despite using ice, then you probably were exercising too strenuously. If the pain persists, then you should contact your physician and discuss what pain is normal and what pain signals something more serious. The things you should alert your doctor to include (1) persistent fatigue or weakness, (2) reduced range of motion of your joints, (3) joint swelling, and (4) continuing or worsening pain.

LET'S GET STARTED: YOUR EXERCISE PROGRAM

Because of your pain, fatigue, and limited joint movement, you are starting this exercise program more deconditioned than your friends without painful joints. But that makes exercise even more important for you, and the sooner you start, the better. Your first steps are to recondition the areas weakened and deconditioned by your arthritis. It's pointless to start a walking program when the muscles supporting your arthritic hips are too weak to support your joints. So first we'll get them strong, and then, we'll get you walking or biking. The most important goal for you isn't to run a marathon (although I'll be the last to discourage you) but to help you engage in your normal activities with minimal pain. You will start with flexibility exercises, giving extra emphasis on the joints that cause you the most pain. I recommend doing the generalized stretching program every day and selecting flexibility exercises from the group that is specific to your painful area(s) for added emphasis. Then after a week or two of working just on flexibility, you should start your weight training program. I have provided you a quick weight training exercise routine that covers all joints. Start with that and make this part of your daily routine just like you have your general flexibility program. You'll feel much better starting your day after you get your blood flowing this way. As you build the muscles supporting your aching joints, you will be better able to tackle the final part of your exercise program, aerobic activity. Because of its repetitive nature (walking is the same movement repeated over and over), it can aggravate arthritic joints. Your aerobic work will help you lose excess body fat and get some of the weight off your aching joints. Think how your poor hips or knees feel hauling around an extra 30 pounds of fat everywhere. I am a big proponent of pool therapy for people with arthritis. There is nothing better for aching joints than to increase their mobility and strength in warm pool water.

You must start slow and increase the duration and intensity of your exercise program over several weeks to months. Progressing too quickly will not allow time for your joints, ligaments, and tendons to adapt to the new stress. Start slow, progress slow. In the first month of your exercise program, you should stop exercising before you reach your limit. This will prevent an exacerbation of your pain and ensure continued success. It is very easy to overdo it the first week as your enthusiasm takes over. But please proceed cautiously. A pain flare will set you back, and I only want you to have success.

Since you have arthritis, the focus of your exercise program will be on muscle strength and flexibility. After your pain is controlled, you should focus on cardio to improve heart health and achieve your optimal weight.

Warm-up for 10 minutes before starting each exercise session. Include the full body stretch routine and specific stretches for your painful joints (found below) at the end of your warm-up session.

Resistance (weight) training for 15–30 minutes 4–5 days a week with special focus on your arthritic areas. Use heavier weights and fewer repetitions to maximize muscle building and minimize joint stress.

Later, add *aerobic exercise* for 10 minutes 3 days a week to start. Then progress to 20–30 minutes, 3 days a week over the next 2–3 months. Start at intensity of 4–5 on the Borg scale if you are new to exercise.

Cooldown for 10 minutes after each session with joint-specific stretching to end your session.

After you are done exercising, it is a good idea to ice your painful joints to reduce swelling and pain. I tell my patients to ice their joints for about 20 minutes after they have finished their cooldown period. Ice for inflammation and by definition arthritis means inflammation of the joints. You will find ice to be a good friend.

WARM-UP (5-10 minutes before every exercise session)

The warm-up period is one of the most important parts of your exercise program because it helps your body prepare for the rigors of exercise and prevents injury. A good warm-up is especially critical to ease aching joints into the rigors of exercise. Start with an easy stroll, and progress to a brisk pace with your arms swinging. This will gradually increase your body temperature and literally warm up your muscles and your joints. Do 10 minutes of walking, followed by 5–10 minutes of stretching. I think the best warm-up is simply walking outside in the fresh air for 10 minutes at a progressively faster pace. By the time the 10 minutes is done, you should be breathing harder and feel that your body is warm.

STRETCHING EXERCISES

After your 5–10 minutes of walking, stretch. These exercises are designed to increase range of motion of your arthritic joints. You may hear popping and cracking at first. This will diminish as you loosen and warm up your joints.

I want the focus of your program to be on your trouble areas. It's hardest to make yourself work the areas that are painful or don't have a good range of motion. But you have to make yourself do the exercises that don't come easy, and pretty soon, it will all be easy and much less painful. Again, a good physical therapist is invaluable to teach you what is safe and ease your fears of injury.

Begin your stretching regimen slowly. You don't need to be able to touch your toes the first day. You will get there. Most important is that when you stretch, you need to use deep breathing to help you relax and hold the stretch. *Do not bounce.* Ever. And once you have finished working out, you should stretch again. Simply repeat the same stretches that you started with.

Before we move to stretches for specific trouble areas, I want to run through a quick stretching session to focus on maintaining full range of motion of all the important joints in your body. This is a great way to start the day, especially after a warm shower has loosened you up. You will be in less pain and more limber the rest of the day.

Sit in a straight-backed chair. You are looking forward with chin in line with your body (not sticking forward), your shoulders back and shoulder blades down, your stomach firm (like you're bracing to be punched in the gut), and your feet on the floor.

1. Turn your head to the side to a count of 2, pause as you look over your shoulder, then return to center. Repeat to the other side. Do this 4–6 times each side.

2. Shrug your shoulders up to your ears as you take a deep breath in. As you let them relax, reach your fingers to the ground and feel a stretch across your shoulders. We all carry so much tension in our shoulders; this is a great exercise to stretch it all away. Repeat 8 times.

3. Now shrug your shoulders again up to your ears, but this time, roll them back and then down in a full shoulder roll. Repeat 8 times.

4. Slowly reach your arms in front of you and bring them up over your head and lower them down in front of you and reach them back behind you and stretch back. Keep your back straight and stomach strong the entire time. Repeat 8 times.

5. Now raise your arms out to the side and lift them up overhead as far as you comfortably can. Slowly lower them. If you can't bring them up over your head, then try each time to raise them a little higher.

6. Bend your arms in front of you at the elbow. Rotate your forearms so that your palms are facing down to the floor. Then rotate them back so your palms face up in the air. Do 8 repetitions in a slow and controlled manner.

7. With your arms still bent at the elbow, bend and flex your wrists 8 times, feeling a good stretch in each direction.

8. Touch the tip of each finger to your thumb. Start with your index finger touching the tip of the finger to your thumb and then open your hand. Repeat with each finger twice and then repeat the whole exercise with the other hand.

9. Slowly raise your right knee to your chest with your hands holding behind your thigh. You must keep your back straight and your stomach strong during this exercise. As you bring your knee to your

chest, pause and then lower your leg. Repeat on the left. Do 8 repetitions on each side.

10. If you have not had a hip replacement, then extend your right leg straight on the ground in front of you. Slowly roll your leg so your toes point inward, and then rotate the whole leg so your toes point out to the side. Repeat 8 times each side and keep your stomach muscles engaged during the entire exercise.

11. With your leg out straight, slowly curl forward to stretch your back and hamstrings. Breathe out as you stretch forward so you can relax into the stretch. No bouncing. As you stretch forward, flex your foot so the toes point up at the ceiling to feel the stretch in your calves. Pause at the end of the stretch and then sit back up.

12. Bend your right knee back, reaching your foot under your chairs far as it will go. Hold for a count of 2, and then straighten your leg and hold it straight out in front of you for a count of 2. Repeat 8 times on the right and then on the left.

13. Ankle circles with your right foot. Rotate your foot clockwise 4 times, and then rotate counterclockwise 4 times. Repeat these big slow circles on the left.

Now it's time to focus on your trouble areas. Below is a selection of stretches for the major trouble areas. These stretches should be part of both your warm-up and cooldown sessions. Remember, the worst thing for an arthritic joint is to lose its flexibility. The focused stretches below are designed to restore the full range of motion to your painful joints. One of the worst-case scenarios is the case of the frozen shoulder. It's a real medical diagnosis and happens when shoulder pain keeps the patient from moving their shoulder. It literally freezes up, and oftentimes even the best physicians and physical therapists can't restore function. So please get those joints moving.

STRETCHES FOR HIPS AND KNEES

Maintaining flexibility of the muscles supporting the hip joint will increase your range of motion and provide agility. It will also improve your balance and help minimize your risk of falling.

ad Stretch

Knee. your right leg bent in front of you with your knee at a 90-degree angle and your left knee on a mat for cushioning. Keep your body vertical, and gently press your hips forward to feel a stretch in the front of the left thigh and hip. Hold for a count of 10, then relax. Repeat 5–10 times and then repeat on the other side.

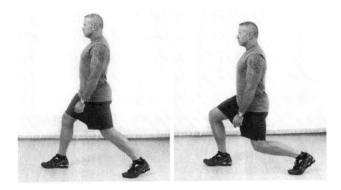

Quadriceps Standing Stretch

Stand facing a chair, holding on to the back lightly for balance. Bend the right knee and grab your ankle with your right hand. Hold for a count of 5, exhaling during the stretch. Try to balance by lifting your hands off the back of the chair on during the stretch to engage core strengthening.

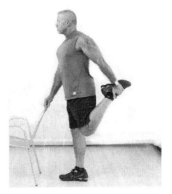

Piriformis Stretch

Lying on your back, bend your right knee with your knee at a 90-degree angle and your foot on the floor. Rest your left ankle on your right leg and let your knee relax out to the side. Gently pull your right knee to your chest and feel the stretch in the left buttock. Hold for a count of 5, exhaling during the stretch.

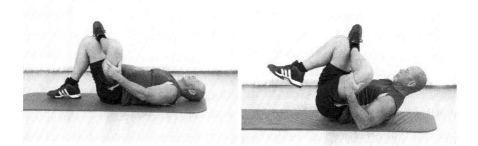

Lateral Hip Wall Stretch

Stand about 1 foot away from the wall with your right forearm resting against the wall. Cross your left leg over the right, keeping your knees straight. Press your right hip toward the wall to feel a stretch along the outside of your right hip. Hold for a count of 5 and exhale during the stretch. Return to your starting position and repeat 5 times on each side.

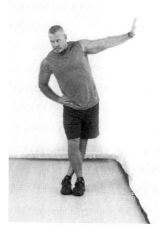

Lying Hamstring Stretch

Lie on your back with both legs straight on the floor and arms by your sides. Bring your right knee to your chest. Place both hands behind your right knee and slowly straighten your right leg. It is OK if you need to lower your right leg to get your knee straight. Hold the straight-leg position for a count of 5, slowly exhaling while you straighten it. Bend the knee again and repeat the exercise 5–10 times on each side.

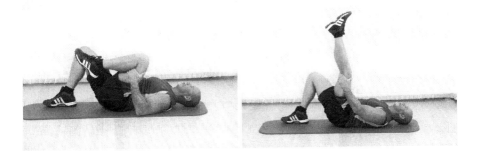

Calf Stretch

Stand on a bottom stair, holding on to the railing for support. Edge your feet back so your heels are off the step. Slowly rise up on your toes and hold for a count of 2. Then lower your body, keeping your knees straight until your heels are below the step and you feel a stretch up the back of your leg.

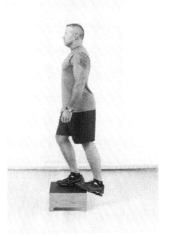

STRETCHES FOR SHOULDERS

Maintaining shoulder flexibility is critical. I know it hurts to move it, but after your doctor has cleared you for exercise, you must maintain your range of motion. Not moving your shoulder can lead to frozen shoulder, known in the medical world as adhesive capsulitis. And once your shoulder is frozen, there is little chance of getting your range of motion back. So start slowly and push just to the limit of pain. You will find that as your joint warms up, you will be able to go a little farther each time.

Raising Shoulder Lying Down

Lie on your back and grab the hand of your painful arm with the other hand. Slowly lift your painful arm up over your head. Repeat 10 times.

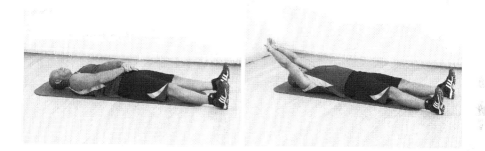

Finger Walk

Stand about a foot away from a smooth wall. Walk your fingers up the wall in front of you until your arm is straight above your head or you are limited by pain. Build yourself up so you can repeat this 10–12 times.

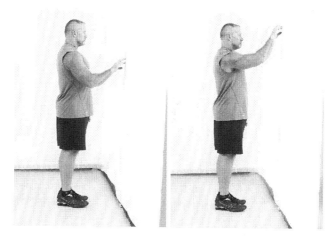

Internal/External Rotation

Stand with your arms at your side. Bend at the elbow with your arm sticking out in front of you. Keeping your elbow by your side, rotate the arm so it lies across your stomach. Return to front and then bend it away from your body. Repeat 12 times.

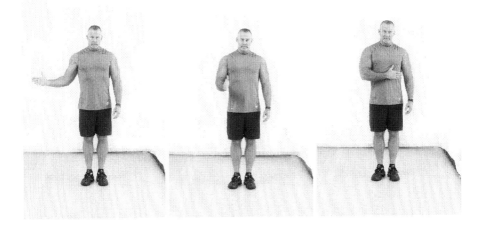

Advanced

Sit in a chair with your back tall and stomach tight. Slowly raise your arms in front of you, and continue lifting till you feel pain or they are up over your head. Breathe in deep as you raise your arms and exhale and you lower them in front of you. Repeat 8 times.

Sit in a chair with your back tall and stomach tight. Slowly raise your arms out to the side and up over your head. Stop when you feel pain, but try with each repetition to reach your arms a little higher over your head. You won't break anything, I promise.

Sit in a chair with your back tall and stomach tight. Raise your right arm and reach behind you to scratch your back. Reach your left arm behind you at waist level and bring the fingers up to meet the fingers of the opposite hand behind your back. Hold for a count of 2 and then switch sides. Repeat 8 times. It's OK if your fingers don't touch behind you, but that is your goal.

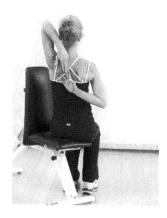

RESISTANCE EXERCISE

The focus of your exercise program is to build strength of the muscles supporting each of your ailing joints without adding unnecessary stress to them. Strong muscles will make daily activities like walking to the car, grocery shopping, or house cleaning that much easier. Weight training will keep your bones strong, and it will also improve your balance. Weight training is also one of the best tools we have to fight fat. And you know those extra pounds you are carrying around are destroying what is left of those painful hips, knees, and back. Weight training increases your muscle mass, and with more muscle, you have a higher resting metabolic rate. That means you are burning more calories with everything that you do. The more muscle you have, the more calories your body is burning even when sitting and watching TV. Muscle is metabolically active tissue—it is burning calories 24 hours a day. Fat just sits there and puts an undue stress on your heart, on your back, and on your joints. As we age and become less active, we lose muscle at an alarming rate. This loss of muscle mass and fall in resting metabolic rate is not an inevitable result of aging. It is a result of our inactivity and sedentary lifestyle. By weight training 3 days a week, you can reverse this loss. Studies have shown that people over the age of 70 can get stronger with a weight training program—you are never too old to start.

Lastly, after you have regained your muscle strength, you will find that your aerobic exercise (whether you chose walking, biking, or swimming) is much easier. In addition, strong muscles will make daily activities like grocery shopping or house cleaning that much easier. Weight training will keep your bones strong, and it will improve your balance. One in three Americans over the age of 65 fall every year, but exercise cannot only improve your balance, but also decreases your risk of falling. But you need to do exercises specifically targeted to your balance problems. For example, if you are unsteady while walking, then exercises that require you balance on one leg will strengthen the muscles you need. I have included a balance training section to help get you started. Please make sure you can do the exercises perfectly on two feet before you try them on one.

To strength train with arthritis, I want you to use weights on the heavy side and limit the number of repetitions you do of each exercise. Using a heavier weight with fewer repetitions is the optimal way to build strength. And by doing fewer repetitions, you will decrease the wear and tear on your joints. Do the exercises in a slow and controlled manner; they are much more difficult and much more effective than fast repetitions, where you rely on momentum to move the weight. In addition, slow, controlled movements are much less stressful on your joints. And moving slowly makes you focus on your form and proper alignment of your spine and maintaining your strong core.

You should start with the beginning program and do 4–6 repetitions of each exercise. So find a weight that allows you to do 6 repetitions with some ease. Each week you should try to increase your number of repetitions of each exercise by 1–2. Once you can easily do 10–12 repetitions of each exercise, increase the weight you lift by 2.5 to 5 lb. Your muscles will adapt much quicker than your joints, so to avoid injury, progress slowly for the first 2 months of your exercise program. If you start noticing pain with your exercise session, then stop or ease back the weight until the pain subsides. Sharp pain that is stronger than your normal arthritic pain is a signal to ease up; lighten the weight and check that you are using the correct form during the exercise.

CORE

Although you'll see everyone in the gym dropping to do 50 sit-ups, they are defeating the purpose on several fronts. The first problem is the number 50. Any exercise you do where you can do more than 20 is not

building strength efficiently. Your best bet is to slow down the
so you recruit more muscle fibers and build strength efficiently.
50 sit-ups does not provide enough muscle resistance to build stren
Working your abs slowly or adding weight will recruit the maxima
number of muscle fibers and provide optimal strength gains. Find 1 or 2
exercises that are hard enough that you can only do 15–20 reps.

The second problem is with the word *sit-up*. It's a bad choice of an
exercise to build core strength. You see, any exercise where you raise
your body up from the floor is using your hip flexor muscles far more
than it uses your abdominal muscles. So with the classic sit-up, you are
training your hip flexors but not your abdominal/core muscles. The sit-up
is not only ineffective, but it is also potentially dangerous. It can easily
strain your low back, a situation we want to avoid. The exercises that
follow are safe for your back and will develop all four of your abdominal
muscles, providing the strong core you need. Your core muscles include
your rectus abdominis muscle, which is your six-pack. But there are
three other sets of muscles that run underneath the rectus muscles.
These three sets of muscles run diagonally and across your belly and
are the ones we want to strengthen. The following exercises focus on
strengthening these. Core also includes your low back muscles. They
work in tandem with your abdominal muscles to provide support for
your back. Pick a combination of exercises from the list below that work
both.

You should do 2–3 of the following exercises as part of your weight
training program. After 4–6 weeks, switch exercises.

Half Locust

Lie on your belly, chin on the floor, arms stretched back alongside your
body with palms down. With your toes pointed, lift your right leg a few
inches off the floor. Hold for several seconds, then slowly lower. Do 3–6
reps; switch legs and repeat (targets back).

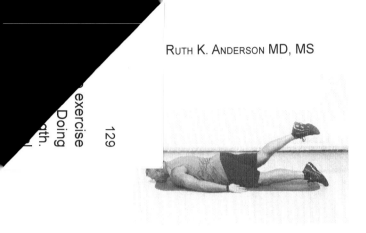

Medicine Ball Twist

Sit on the floor with your legs extended and your back straight. Place a medicine ball (start with a light ball) next to your right hip. Twist and pick up the ball and place it beside the opposite hip. Repeat on each side for a total of 12–15 reps.

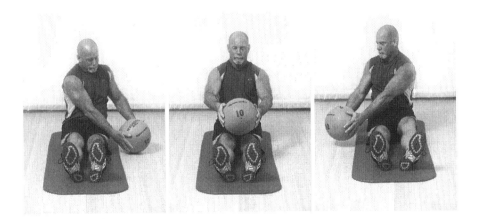

Resistance One-Leg Crunch

Lie on your back with your knees bent with your feet on the floor. Lift your right knee and resist the movement with your right arm. Hold for a count of 2 and then return to the starting position. Repeat on the left. That is 1 repetition. Work up so you can do 8–12 reps (targets abs).

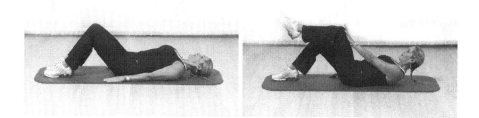

Pelvic Tilt

On the floor, lie on your back with your knees bent. Your feet are flat on the floor and your arms at your sides, palms facing the ground. To a count of 2, slowly roll your pelvis so that hips and lower back are off the floor while upper back and shoulders remain in place. Hold for a count of 2, then slowly lower. Repeat 10 times (targets back, glutes, and abs).

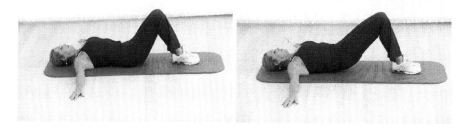

My Crunch

Lie on the floor; with fingers lightly behind your ears, slowly raise your shoulders and buttocks at the same time. If you are doing the exercise correctly, then you will feel your lower abdominal muscles along with your six-pack engage. It is more important to try to lift your buttocks off the floor than lift your shoulders. Hold for 2 seconds and slowly return to your starting position. Do as many as you can with perfect form (targets abs).

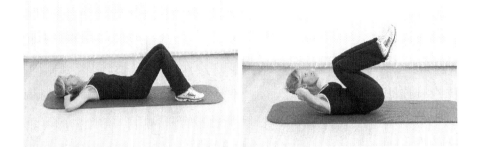

Superman

This works your back extensor muscles with minimal stress on your spine compared to more traditional back exercises.

Kneel on your hands and knees. Keep your stomach tight (like you're being punched), but keep the normal arch in your lower back. Straighten your right leg behind you, keeping it at hip level. Then raise your right arm so it extends straight out at ear level. Keep both your outstretched arm and leg parallel to the floor. Hold for a count of 4, then repeat on the other side. Do 6–8 repetitions each side (lower back, glutes, and hamstrings).

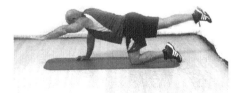

When that becomes simple, start from a standard push-up position and raise your left leg while maintaining the perfect push-up position (targets abdominals, back, hamstrings, and glutes).

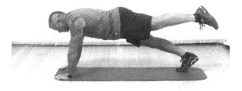

Plank

This is one of my favorite core-strengthening exercises.

Assume a modified push-up position with your forearms resting on the floor. Elbows should be under your shoulders and bent at 90 degrees. Keep your torso steady and your body in a straight line from your head to your toes. Do not let your stomach sag. Hold for as long as you can. Your goal is to hold this for 30 seconds (targets abs and back).

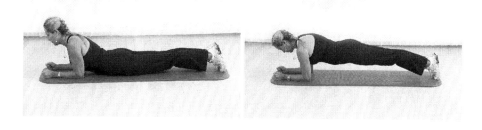

FOR ARTHRITIC KNEES

Start with isometric exercises to build muscle strength. These are exercises where you contract your muscles but don't move your leg or arm.

Sitting Knee Extension (isometric)

Sit on a chair facing a wall. Sit close to the wall. Rest your foot against the wall and push forward. Hold for a count of 5. Repeat 3–5 times and then do the same thing on the left (targets quadriceps).

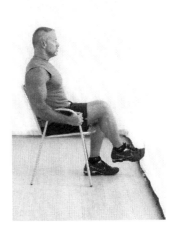

After you can do this exercise easily without flaring your knee pain, begin the following strengthening program. Pick 2–3 exercises from the following list to start with. After 4–6 weeks, when they become easy, add a new exercise to your routine. Do each exercise slowly and watch your form carefully. Keep your stomach strong (tense it like you're going to be punched in the gut) and knees over your toes. The slower you do the exercises, the more muscle fibers you will recruit—a fancy way of saying that you will work harder.

After you can do all these exercises easily without flaring your pain, you need to try doing them faster. Since muscle training is very specific, if you only train with slow motions, then your muscles will be strong only when you move slowly. Yet we need to be able to move quickly at times (e.g., crossing the street before the light changes or catching our balance so we don't fall). So once you know how to do the exercises safely at a slow pace, pick it up. Try moving faster during at least 1 exercise session each week.

Sit to Stand

Sit on a firm straight-backed chair. Engage your core (tighten your stomach like someone was going to punch you in the gut). With stomach strong, slowly stand up. Use your legs, not your arms, to lift your body off the chair. If you cannot stand without using your arms, then allow them to assist you—but no more than necessary. Slowly lower back to the seated position, but halfway down, pause for a count of 2 or 4, then continue to the seated position. Do as many as you can with perfect form (targets quadriceps, core).

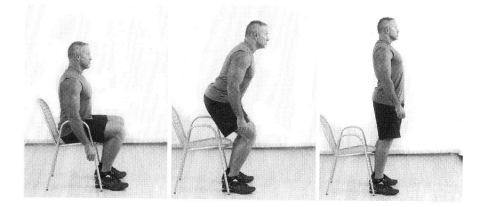

Seated Leg Extension

Sit in a firm straight-backed chair with knees bent and feet on the floor. Slowly extend your right leg until it is straight out in front of you. Hold your leg in the straight position for a count of 4, then lower. When you can do this, slightly raise your leg off the chair once you have straightened it. Keep your back straight and your stomach firm and hold your leg off the chair for a count of 2–4, then lower your leg and return to the starting position. Do 10–12 reps with each leg. When it gets easy, lift your leg higher (targets quadriceps).

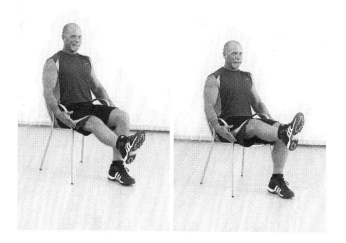

Step Up

Stand straight with your stomach strong. Step your right foot onto first step and slowly straighten leg. Keep toes facing front. Bring left foot up to touch step by right ankle, then slowly lower your weight to count of 4 onto left leg. Don't push off back leg. Move slowly so the muscles, and not the momentum, do the work. As you stand up, press your weight through the heel, not the ball, of your foot. Do 15–20 reps with each leg. When the stair step becomes easy, carry 5–10 lb. dumbbells to increase difficulty (targets quadriceps and glutes, balance).

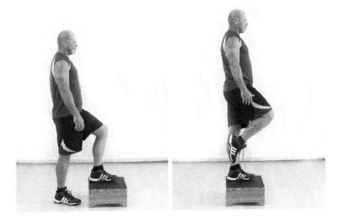

Wall Squat

Stand with a fitness ball between you and a wall. Rest your lower back against the fitness ball. Your feet should be shoulder width apart and about 3 feet away from the wall. Slowly bend your knees till your thighs are parallel to the floor, or as low as you can go. Make sure you keep your knees directly over your toes. Pause and then squeeze your buttocks as you return to the standing position. Build up to 10 repetitions. As this gets easier, deepen your knee bend to optimize quadriceps strengthening (targets quadriceps, glutes).

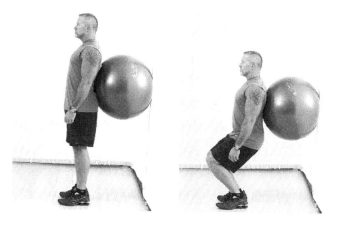

FOR ARTHRITIC HIPS

Pick 2–3 exercises from the following list. After 4–6 weeks, when they become easy, add a new exercise to your routine. Do each exercise slowly and watch your form carefully. Keep your stomach strong (tense it like you're going to be punched in the gut) and knees over your toes. The slower you do the exercises, the more muscle fibers you will recruit—a fancy way of saying that you will work harder. After you can do all these exercises easily without flaring your pain, you need to try doing them quickly. Since muscle training is very specific, if you only train with slow motions, then your muscles will be strong only when you move slowly. Yet we need to be able to move quickly at times (e.g., crossing the street before the light changes or catching our balance so we don't fall). So once you know how to do the exercises safely at a slow pace, pick it up. Try moving faster during at least 1 of your exercise sessions a week.

Hip Abduction

Stand facing a chair. With your arms on the back of a chair for balance, slowly raise your right leg out to the side and hold for a count of 2. Lower and repeat with the left leg. As it gets easy, increase the height you lift your leg, and don't hold on. Work up to 12 reps on each side (targets hip abductors, balance).

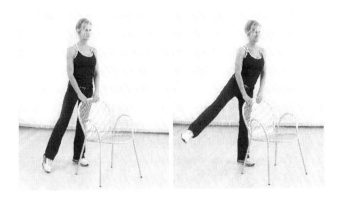

Standing Hip Flexion

Stand next to a chair with your feet together and hold on to the chair with your left hand for support. Bend your right knee and lift it up to your waist, pause, and slowly lower it. Repeat 8 times and then turn and do the same thing with the left leg. When this gets easy, do it without holding on to your leg (targets hip flexors, balance).

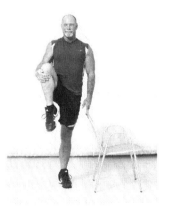

Kneeling Leg Lift

Kneel on your hands and knees with your arms under your shoulders and knees under your hips. Keep your core strong or abdominal muscles pulled tight so there is a straight line from your head to your hips. Extend your right leg out to the side. Lift your leg to hip height and move it in a semicircle, crossing it behind you and touching your toes to the ground on the outside of your left leg. Build up to 8–12 repetitions on each leg (targets glutes, abductors).

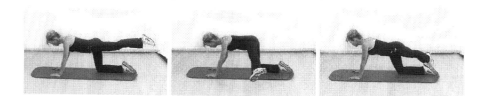

Hip Bridge

Lying on your back with heels tucked close to your buttocks, lift your buttocks off the ground so your body forms a straight line from knees to shoulders. Hold for 2 seconds, then slowly lower over a 2-second count. Do 8–12 reps (targets hamstrings, glutes, and low back).

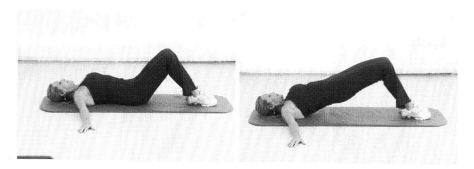

For added difficulty, straighten your right leg from the knee and do the movement using only the left leg to lift your body. Keep the right leg straight during the exercise. Do 8–12 reps on each side.

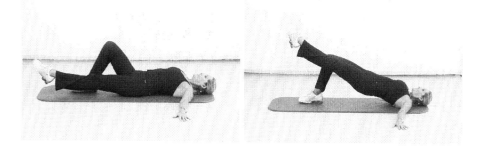

For even more difficulty, straighten your right leg with your toes pointing at the ceiling. Keep your leg pointed toward the ceiling as you raise your body with your left leg. Do 8–12 reps, then repeat with the left leg straight.

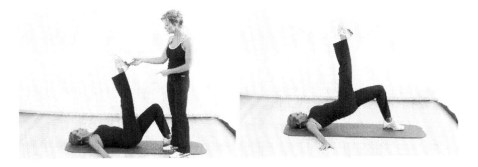

Fire Hydrant

Kneel on all fours on a mat and place a 1 or 3 lb. weight behind your right knee. Squeeze your leg muscles so that the dumbbell stays locked in place. Keeping your back flat and your head down, slowly raise your right leg until your thigh is parallel with the floor. Pause and then lower your right leg to the starting position. Do 8–12 reps on each side (targets hamstrings and glutes).

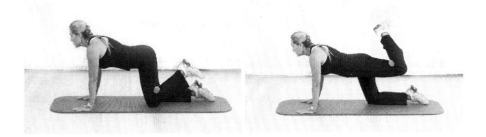

Dumbbell Split Squat

Step your right foot forward about 12 inches and your left leg back about 12 inches. Keep your chest up and stomach tight, bend both knees, and lower your body to a slow count of 4 and then straighten your legs to the same slow count. Stop when your form begins to slip. Do 6–15 reps.

For added difficulty, hold your arms over your head or hold 5–10 lb. dumbbells at your sides (targets quadriceps, hamstrings, and glutes, balance).

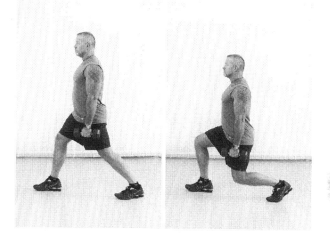

BALANCE

Many of the exercises presented in this chapter, or any other chapter for that matter, can also incorporate balance training. But these are specifically designed to give you a good starting point for balance training. It is another one of those areas that if you don't *move it*, then you will *lose it*. You must practice balance just as you practice your golf swing. When these become simple, then you can start doing any exercise on one leg to continue to challenge yourself. In addition, daily balance practice is easy to incorporate into your daily routine. Just brush your teeth on one leg or brush them with your eyes closed.

Eyes Closed

Stand on a thick folded towel with your feet shoulder width apart. Stand tall with your abdominal muscles engaged (say *sshhh* to engage them). Close your eyes and visualize the upright position.

Balance on One Leg

Stand with your hand on a chair or bar for support. Shift your weight to your left leg and lift the right leg off the floor. Try letting go of your support or only resting your fingertips on the bar for balance. Your goal is to stand on one leg for 30 seconds. Turn around and repeat it standing on your right leg.

Marching in Place

Stand tall with your core strong (say *sshhh* to engage your abdominal muscles). March in place slowly, lifting your knees as high as you can. When this is easy, do it on a folded towel or soft cushion.

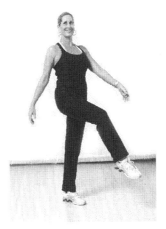

Eyes Closed

Stand on a thick folded towel with your feet shoulder width apart. Stand tall with your abdominal muscles engaged (say 'Shhh' to engage them). Close your eyes and visualize the upright position.

Balance On One Leg

Stand with your hand on a chair or bar for support. Shift your weight to your left leg and lift the right leg off the floor. Try letting go of your support or only resting your finger tips on the bar for balance. You goal is to stand on one leg for 30 seconds. Turn around and repeat it standing on your right leg.

Advanced

Fold a bath towel several times over, place it on the floor, and stand on the center of the towel. This will give you a slightly unstable surface because the towel is soft.

Advanced

Try doing the one-leg balance with your eyes shut. Keep the chair back close so you can steady yourself as needed.

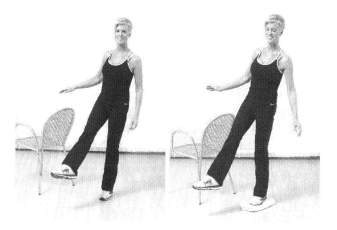

Toe-Stand Balance

Stand facing a sturdy chair or bar with your hands resting lightly on it. Rise up onto your toes and try to let go of the chair and balance for a count of 10. When you are an expert, raise up on your toes and, still holding on gently, shift your weight to the right leg and try to balance on your toes on one leg. You will feel the muscles of your entire leg and your core engage. Keep your head high and stomach strong (say *sshhh*).

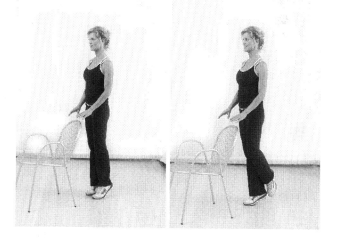

FOR ARTHRITIC SHOULDERS

Shoulders are especially susceptible to injury due to the anatomy of the joint. If you are having shoulder pain that limits your ability to raise your arms, scratch your back, or blow-dry your hair, then I recommend that you start with a physical therapist to learn how to strengthen your rotator cuff muscles properly. The rotator cuff muscles provide stability to your shoulder joint. Once these muscles are strong, you can proceed with the exercises I have included here.

You will notice that all the exercises in this section are done with free weights. I strongly suggest that you avoid using weight lifting machines for your shoulders. They can aggravate the problem instead of help it.

Pick 2–3 exercises from the following list to start with. After 4–6 weeks, when they become easy, add a new exercise to your routine. Do each exercise slowly and watch your form carefully. Keep your stomach strong (tense it like you're going to be punched in the gut) and knees over your toes. The slower you do the exercises, the more muscle fibers you will recruit—a fancy way of saying that you will work harder.

Shoulder Shrug

Stand holding a 3–5 lb. dumbbell in each hand, palms facing toward each other. Shrug your shoulders up to your ears and pause. Slowly lower your shoulders. Repeat 12 times (targets shoulders).

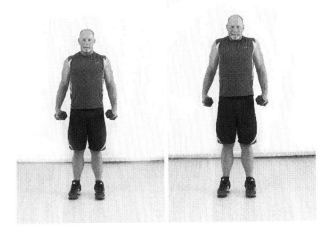

Shoulder Raise

Sit on a bench holding a 1 or 3 lb. weight. Raise the weight out to the side until your arm is at a 90-degree angle at the shoulder or you have pain. Slowly bring the weight to the front, keeping your arm at the same

90-degree height. Repeat on the other side. Do 12–15 reps each side. When your shoulder feels stable with the 1 lb. weight, you can step up to a heavier weight. You can also do this exercise standing to engage your core muscles for a double benefit (targets shoulders).

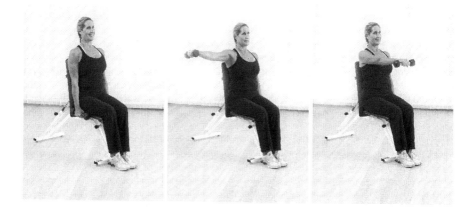

Controlled Fly

Kneel on a bench with your right leg and right arm on the bench. In your left hand, you are holding a 1 or 3 lb. weight with the palm facing you. Keep your back flat and stomach strong during the exercise. Slowly lift the weight out to the side till your arm is parallel to the floor. Repeat 10 times with each arm (targets shoulders).

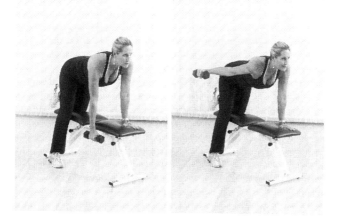

Toss and Catch

Play toss and catch with a beach ball or light medicine ball. As the exercise gets easier, you can increase the weight of the ball. Keep your stomach engaged (tense the muscles like you're going to be punched in the stomach) throughout your game, especially right before you throw the ball (targets shoulders and abs).

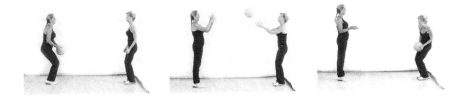

Internal Rotation

Lie on a bench with the weak side down and the elbow bent at a right angle. Hold the dumbbell in your weak hand. Curl the weight in toward your abdomen. Repeat 20 times. As this gets easier, increase the weight of the dumbbell (targets shoulder rotator cuff muscles).

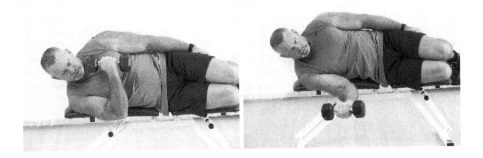

External Rotation

Lie on your side on a bench with your top arm flat against your side. Hold a 1–3 lb. weight in your upper hand and bend your elbow so your hand and forearm are pointing forward. Keep your elbow next to your side and rotate the dumbbell up into the air so your forearm and hand point toward the ceiling. You won't be able to go the whole way vertical—just 45 degrees or so (targets shoulder rotator cuff muscles).

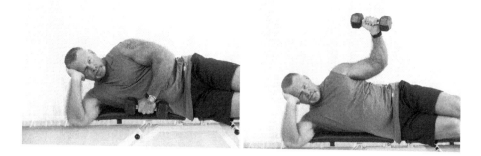

Incline Press

Lie on an incline bench with a light dumbbell in each hand, elbows bent, and the weights resting beside your chest. With palms facing each other, slowly push the weights toward the ceiling until your shoulder blade comes off the bench. Slowly lower the weights to the starting position. Repeat 10 times. When this becomes easy, increase the weight of the dumbbells (targets shoulders and chest).

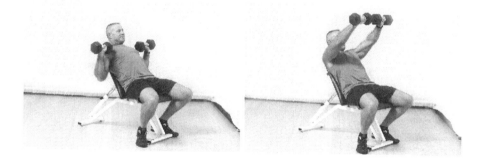

AEROBIC EXERCISE (10–30 minutes 3 days a week)

Aerobic exercise will be the last step in your exercise program. You can begin this when you have developed enough joint flexibility and muscle strength to tolerate the repetitive movement of aerobic exercise. After doing the resistance exercises described above for several weeks, you should see an improvement in your ability to move your aching joint(s). That is when it's time to add some total body conditioning to your exercise program—cardio. Your heart, lungs, and muscles deserve some strengthening and conditioning too. Choose any activity that you enjoy and are comfortable doing. Remember, these are the -ing words, and they include walking, hiking, biking, and swimming (I recommend that you avoid running to be gentle to your joints). Swimming and pool aerobics in a warm pool are especially beneficial for arthritis sufferers. But if you are uncomfortable in a bathing suit, then pool exercise is not for you—find what *you* enjoy. And adapt your exercise to your pain. When it hurts, stop. You will have some discomfort, but before it gets to be pain, you need to stop. Over the days and weeks to come, you will find you can do much more exercise before the pain stops you.

Opt for more intense activities that move your joints slower. For example, when you bike (stationary or street), increase the pedal resistance so you pedal harder but move your legs slower. Avoid spinning classes, which wear out arthritic joints. Walk up hills or take stairs (as your knees tolerate) rather than walk on flat ground. This will work your muscles harder, increase your heart rate, and at the same time, save your joints.

COOLDOWN (5-10 minutes after every exercise session)

The cooldown is important to minimize muscle soreness and fatigue. During exercise, your body accumulates lactic acid (a by-product of muscle work). We associate lactic acid buildup with muscle soreness. The cooldown period gives your body a chance to clear the lactic acid from your muscles and minimizes postworkout discomfort. Do not stop exercising abruptly. If you simply stop after exercising vigorously, then there is a good chance your blood pressure will drop and you will get light-headed and dizzy. Keep moving. It's what all the experts say and for very good reason. Especially if you have any history of coronary artery disease, then you need to make the cooldown period an important priority. Think of the cooldown period as "active rest," where you are gently returning your body to its pre-exercise state.

Walk slowly for about 10 minutes after you finish exercising to gently return your heart rate to its resting level. Or you can simply do a slower version of whatever exercise you were doing. Continue walking until you are breathing normally and can easily carry on a conversation. During your cooldown period is the best time to stretch. But wait until your heart rate has slowed and is approaching your resting rate.

Take advantage of your joints' increased temperature and suppleness and do the majority of your stretching right after you have finished your active cooldown.

I listed all the stretching exercises in the warm-up section to get your attention and help you focus on their importance. But flexibility gains are best made when your muscles are warm, and that occurs after your exercise session. So go back to the warm-up section and start stretching. Use this cooldown time for overall body stretching and for maintaining flexibility of your specific arthritic joints.

I believe the wise men who say that we are masters of our own fate. Our life is ours, our health is ours, our happiness is ours. Once you take responsibility for your health, you have the power to change it. Stop blaming, stop complaining, and slowly, with love and tenderness, pick yourself up off the couch and go for your first walk. It is the walk of your lifetime.

The Arthritis Foundation is doing an amazing job at providing information on the disease and its treatments. They also offer several community-based exercise programs for individuals with arthritis. I strongly encourage you to contact them. There is so much you can do for yourself, and they will help.

EXERCISE TO TREAT DIABETES

Diabetes (type 2 or adult-onset diabetes) is one disease that you can control, even obliterate, with a regular exercise program coupled with weight loss. Think about it. You have the power within you to cure this disease. As a doctor, I can't cure your disease. I can give you medicine to control your symptoms, but that medicine doesn't cure your diabetes. However, when you take responsibility for your disease, you have the power to control your blood sugar through weight loss and exercise and actually stop your medication.

Type 2 diabetes, also called non-insulin-dependent diabetes, occurs when the cells of your body become resistant to the effects of insulin. Because insulin can't do its job, your body can't regulate your blood sugar and your blood sugar rises. Elevated blood sugar causes damage to many organ systems, resulting in an increased chance of heart disease, kidney failure, stroke, liver disease, blindness, and damage to peripheral nerves leading to severe pain called diabetic peripheral neuropathy.

With regular—and I mean regular—exercise, you will help your body handle the carbohydrates/sugar that you eat and enable your body to process the sugar so it can't damage your organs. The exercise impact I'm referring to works for adult-onset diabetes, but it can also improve glucose control in type 1 or juvenile-onset diabetes as well. My focus here is on adult-onset diabetes. We know that it's the highly refined carbohydrate load in our processed foods (bread, cakes, ice cream) that is the biggest cause of elevated blood sugar in people with diabetes. And it's the sugar that circulates through your bloodstream that wreaks havoc on your organs. It takes very little sugar in your bloodstream to cause all this damage. Normally you have about a teaspoon of sugar circulating in your blood. The difference between a man who has diabetes and one who doesn't is only about one-fourth teaspoon of sugar. That's all we have to control—that measly little one-fourth teaspoon.

We know that along with diet, exercise is one of the most important things anyone can do to treat their disease. It's one of the cheapest and easiest. Doctors know how important exercise is. They tell every one of their patients to get exercising. But although doctors know a lot about your disease, we don't have a quick, easy answer to your question "So how do I start?" or "What do I do?" Well, here you go. Here is your start. The following is a guided program to start you on a safe and effective program to change your life and treat your disease.

WHY EXERCISE?

Exercise, both endurance (cardio) and resistance (weight training), is too often an underutilized therapy to treat diabetes. Every diabetic should be on a regular exercise routine. Exercise improves your body's ability to process the sugar/carbohydrates that you eat, and the benefits last for up to 72 hours after your last exercise session. So to continue to reap the benefits of your exercise program, you should exercise every other day. That's not bad. I appreciate that diabetes is a very regimented disease requiring you to continually monitor what you eat and check your blood sugars on a regular basis. And here I am asking you to add one more scheduled activity into your life. I understand your rebellion. What I don't understand is your refusal to begin an exercise and weight loss program that gives you the power to beat this disease. Weight loss and exercise give you the power to put those pills and your glucometer in the back of your closet. If you are a type 2 diabetic, then you can actually win. You can eradicate this disease. There are several ways exercise fights diabetes.

With exercise, your body's blood sugar is lowered not only during but also after each exercise session—for 72 hours. In addition, with regular exercise and weight loss, your body again becomes more sensitive to insulin so it can do its job better at keeping your blood sugar low. Exercise will also help you lose weight, which will dramatically improve your body's ability to handle the carbohydrates/sugar that you eat. Do you remember when you were thin? You didn't have diabetes then. Your disease is a choice you made. Not consciously, but by making certain lifestyle choices, many of you picked your disease. Now it's time to unpick it. Now you have a choice to not have the disease any longer. Diet and exercise together have the greatest chance to cure your diabetes. Every doctor knows this. But it's up to you to put it into effect.

Now as you continue your exercise program, you will find that the scales lie. They lie about the changes that are happening in your body. As you begin exercising, you will be increasing your muscle mass. But you must remember that muscle weighs more than fat. So you may find that the scale isn't budging, or even worse, you are gaining weight as you increase your muscle mass. I tell my patients to watch their waistline. The scale may not change, but you will find the inches melting away (because, of course, you are watching your calorie intake as well). Scales lie. They don't reflect the changes in your body composition as you burn off fat and put on heavier muscle. The scales lie, but your mirror doesn't.

BEFORE YOU BEGIN

Before starting any exercise program, you should get clearance from your doctor. Sounds familiar, I know. But it is much more than a way for me to cover my legal behind. Having diabetes significantly increases your risk of having heart disease. And because diabetes messes with your nervous system (hence, peripheral neuropathy), the warning signs of heart disease, like chest pain, are not always present. So a pre-exercise evaluation is critical for your safety. Actually, it's critical whether you're exercising or not. Your physician may want you to have a stress test to evaluate your heart function before starting on your own. It is a very good idea. A resting ECG (electrocardiogram, which gives a picture of how your heart is functioning) only gives us a picture of your heart when it is at rest—not under stress. To exercise safely on your own, your doctor needs to see how your heart performs under the stress of exercise. This will unmask problems that aren't evident otherwise. Because of your risk for "silent heart disease," you should get clearance from your doctor before starting *any* exercise program. And if you have heart disease, then you must start slowly and under your physician's direction. While you are waiting for your doctor's appointment, I encourage you to start your walking program. Light activity is the perfect way to start and is not associated with increased cardiac risk. In fact, that is how I will tell you to start your program anyway.

The good news is that exercise lowers your risk of heart disease, so starting your exercise program will benefit you on many levels (or kill many birds with that one exercising-physically-fit stone).

SAFETY PRECAUTIONS

Diabetics have two unique risks that we have to discuss before you can safely start your exercise program. One is the presence of diabetic peripheral neuropathy, and the second is the risk of falling blood sugar with exercise:

1. Diabetic peripheral neuropathy increases your risk for undetected blisters and sores developing on your feet. This is because your elevated blood sugar has destroyed the nerves in your feet, the nerves that would normally sense pain and discomfort. Patients with peripheral neuropathy don't feel what other people feel because their nerves no longer work well. Therefore, you must visually inspect your feet often to catch blisters and treat them appropriately. Another problem that accompanies diabetes is poor blood flow. And if your blood isn't flowing well, then your blisters won't heal. So be vigilant. And please wear good shoes and cushioned socks. Pick sneakers with good support and ample toe room.

Peripheral neuropathy also makes balance more challenging because you don't have the normal feedback from the nerves in your feet. Adjusting to uneven terrain and bumps in the road during your walk is an extra challenge for you. Catching your foot on the edge of the sidewalk could mean a big fall if your peripheral neuropathy makes a quick adjustment in your stride impossible. If you have peripheral neuropathy, then I recommend walking indoors at a mall where you can walk on a smooth surface and can avoid falls. There are no bumps in the sidewalk at the mall.

2. Your second concern as a diabetic is a drop in blood sugar during or after exercise. Although we want the glucose-lowering effects of exercise, we don't want your blood sugar to drop so low you have symptoms like light-headedness or dizziness. Hypoglycemia or low

blood sugar can happen during or after exercise. If your blood sugar drops too low, then you may feel shaky, anxious, sweat more, or notice a change in your heart rate. So while exercising, have a snack handy like an apple, raisins, or a piece of candy. We do want the glucose-lowering effects of exercise, but I don't want it to get too low. When starting an exercise program, you should check your blood sugar before and after your workout. If you haven't eaten in an hour or your blood sugar is less than 120, then eat or drink something before you exercise. You will soon learn how much you can exercise before you start to get hypoglycemic. What is most exciting is that with a regular exercise program and weight loss, you and your doctor will have to decrease your diabetic medication as your body is better able to manage its blood sugar levels on its own.

DIABETIC PERIPHERAL NEUROPATHY—A SPECIAL EXERCISE BENEFIT

Diabetic peripheral neuropathy is often associated with severe chronic pain in your extremities. This pain is a burning, fire, knifelike type of pain that results from damage to the nerves in your arms and legs from the high levels of sugar circulating in your blood. Regular exercise not only helps control your blood sugar, but it is also one of the most effective treatments we have for chronic pain conditions. Generally, patients with chronic pain like diabetic peripheral neuropathy show significant improvement in aerobic conditioning after starting an exercise program. And these improvements are seen within as little as 4 weeks of training. In addition to aerobic exercise, I will give you exercises to improve your balance and strength to combat the negative impact of peripheral neuropathy on your balance.

Patients in pain often decrease their level of physical activity because they are afraid that movement will worsen their pain and that exercise, because it hurts, is signaling that they are making their disease worse. Unfortunately, the opposite is true. Chronic pain, like the pain of diabetic peripheral neuropathy or low back pain, gets worse with inactivity. The normal response for patients with diabetic peripheral neuropathy is to become less active as they avoid all activities that cause pain. We naturally think that if walking hurts or exercising hurts, then we shouldn't do it. But with chronic pain disease, pain is not a signal of tissue damage. It serves no function. It just hurts. It hurts because your diabetes has destroyed your nerves, and all they know how to do after being destroyed is to hurt. As a patient with chronic pain, you must begin exercising. Exercise to treat your diabetes and exercise to treat your pain.

If your diabetic peripheral neuropathy is severe, then I recommend starting your program with the supervision of a physical therapist. Your doctor will write you a prescription for this. Start slow, use pain as your guideline for when to stop, and slowly you will see that if done gently with a very gradual progression that no harm is being done. Your pain is a disease, not a warning signal of damage. Most importantly, you will see your pain improve. The way the body heals itself is by circulating blood to damaged tissues and diseased areas of the body. Exercise increases blood flow. Blood carries oxygen to these damaged areas for healing and carries away toxic waste products. You will never heal by sitting on the couch watching TV. You will heal through exercise.

Now you are ready. You are armed with knowledge and infused with enthusiasm. You can do this. And knowing what I have taught you, you can do it well. Your exercise time will be well spent because I will tell you where to focus your energy to meet your specific goals. The most important thing is that you just need to get started.

LET'S GET STARTED: YOUR EXERCISE PROGRAM

A well-rounded exercise program includes four components: aerobic exercise, strength training, balance, and flexibility. Since you have diabetes, the focus of your exercise program will be on blood sugar control and weight loss—that is achieved most effectively with aerobic exercise. After you start, you will find that your heart gets stronger and healthier and your cholesterol and triglyceride levels are improved. In addition, your stress levels are lower and your libido is stronger. Shall I go on?

Here is the outline of your exercise program:

Warm-up for 10 minutes before starting each exercise session.

Aerobic exercise for 10 minutes 3 days a week initially, then progress over the next 2 months to 30–40 minutes 4 to 5 days a week. If you are new to exercise, then start at a 4–5 level intensity on the perceived exertion scale and work up to 5–6 intensity level.

Resistance (weight) training for 15 to 30 minutes 3–4 days a week to supplement your aerobic work. Your goal is to do 12–20 reps of 1–2 exercises from each section.

Cooldown for 10–15 minutes after each session.

These are your guidelines. The most important thing you can do is learn to listen to your body and adapt your exercise intensity and duration to its needs. If your knees are hurting during exercise and continue to hurt for several hours after you're done, then that is a signal that you pushed too hard and need to slow down the next session. If you are no longer winded during your exercise session, then that is a signal that your body is getting stronger and you need to pick up your pace to continue to provide an exercise challenge. If you are exercising and just don't have the energy or the drive to continue, then listen to your body and stop for the day. Pat yourself on the back for the work that you have done and go home. You can work harder the next time. Remember, you don't have to be an aerobic animal every day to make significant progress. But you do need to listen to your body and respect what it is telling you. On the flip side, if you just don't feel like exercising, then go for a 10-minute walk. Just get yourself off the couch and move. I'll bet once you get going, your walk time turns from 10 minutes to 30 minutes. But if it doesn't, then still pat yourself on the back for overcoming your resistance and taking a positive step for yourself.

WARM-UP (10 to 15 minutes before every exercise session)

The warm-up period is one of the most important parts of your exercise program because it helps your body prepare for the rigors of exercise and prevents injury.

Start with an easy walk that progresses to a brisk pace with your arms swinging. This will gradually increase your body temperature and literally warm up your muscles and your joints. You want to get your blood flowing and your heart pumping. As you warm up, you will warm up your muscles, tendons, and ligaments, which will help prevent injury.

AEROBIC EXERCISE (30-40 minutes 4-5 days a week)

So you have been cleared by your doctor to start an exercise program. And in all his wisdom, he recommends starting with a walking program. I agree 100%. For those of you just starting out, you should exercise only 10–15 minutes a day. Your goal for heart health and weight loss is eventually 30–40 minutes 5 days a week. Find what you enjoy. Walking, biking, hiking, rowing, dancing are all very good aerobic activities. Even gardening and vacuuming are aerobic if you increase your heart rate and are breathing heavy for 30 minutes.

Start your exercise program by walking 10–15 minutes 5 days a week. That's it. You will soon find that a 15-minute stroll is not enough of a challenge, and you will naturally increase your pace. You must not only exercise your muscles, but you must also exercise some patience. Your muscles will adapt fairly quickly to the demands of your new exercise program. And they will adapt much quicker than your ligaments, tendons, and joints. That's where the injuries usually occur. Gradually increase your exercise duration so that all body tissues have time to strengthen and adapt. It's too easy to overdo it and let an injury derail all your good intentions. Patience and gradual progress are much harder to accept but are the only way for lasting success. Start an intensity of about 4–5 on the perceived exertion scale (definitely exercising but at a comfortable place where you can maintain a conversation easily). Your intensity goal is a 5–6 on the scale (breathing heavily but you can still chat with your exercise partner). To optimize fat burning, you want to exercise a little easier so you can exercise longer. This will optimize fat burning—remember, it's the fat that is causing your type 2 diabetes. Aerobic exercise for 30–40 minutes 4–5 days a week is optimal for fat burning (as long as you don't reward yourself with a muffin after every exercise session). It took you time to put on the fat, and it will take a time commitment to get it off. But I promise, it will come off. It is very easy to overestimate the calories you burn during exercise and increase the amount you eat as a reward. Don't or you will defeat your purpose. And definitely never believe the calorie readout on the machines at the gym. They lie. Cut the number in half and you're getting closer to calorie-burn reality. For fat loss, remember, portion control is your best ally.

That is the prescription for health and weight loss for diabetics. The only tough part is to make the commitment and stick with it. But as I see it, you don't have a choice. Your body is screaming as loud as it can that it can't survive the life you have chosen. It is getting sicker by the day. So let's choose health and literally take the first steps on the right track. If you have been totally sedentary, then you will see significant benefits if you start with even a slow stroll. Just start. Remember, the goal is to make a commitment to yourself that you can keep. There is an enormous amount of hype about when you exercise or what kind of exercise you do. But the only important thing is that you *just do it.*

All you need to do is find what works for you and be proud of every baby step you take because each step is a step toward success.

RESISTANCE EXERCISES (15–30 minutes 3–4 days a week)

Weight training should not be the primary focus of your exercise routine. Spend the majority of your time doing aerobic work. It is your ticket to fat burning. But as a tool to increase your muscle mass and increase your metabolic rate, there is nothing better than resistance work to facilitate weight loss. If you have other problems like low back pain or arthritis, then please read that chapter and adjust your weight training according to the recommendations in that chapter. The exercises I have selected here are for people with no painful physical limitations. These exercises are designed to use a number of muscle groups at a time to optimize the efficiency of your weight training session and increase your calorie burn. Select 1–2 exercises from each group to provide a complete full-body workout. You should try to do 12–20 reps with perfect form for each exercise. That means picking a weight that is heavy enough that you can barely do 20 reps, but one that is light enough you can easily do more than 12. Additional exercises are given so you can change your routine every 4–6 weeks.

Once you are a pro and can do all these exercises safely and with perfect form, I want you to take them onto a balance board like a BOSU board. This will add a new dimension of difficulty and stress and strengthen your muscles even more.

A second way to up your intensity is to add a pause during the exercise. For example, pause halfway down during your push-up, hold for 2 seconds, and then continue the movement. The way to continue to improve is by making changes in your exercise program that continue to stress your muscles. Stay out of your comfort zone and find ways to mix up your exercise routine.

LEGS AND GLUTES

Pick one exercise from each of the leg sections: glutes, hamstrings, and calves. The exercises in these sections have good overlap, so you'll be working the same muscles several ways, just with a different focus in each grouping. Start with just one exercise per group and later increase the number to continue to challenge your muscles. Pick a new exercise every 4–6 weeks. And don't forget the balance exercises at the end of this section.

LEGS–QUADS

Sit to Stand

Sit on a firm straight-backed chair. Engage your core (tighten your stomach like someone was going to punch you in the gut). With stomach strong, slowly stand up. Use your legs, not your arms, to lift your body off the chair. If you cannot stand without using your arms, then allow them to assist you—but no more than necessary. Slowly lower back to the seated position, but halfway down, pause for a count of 2 or 4, then continue to the seated position. Do as many as you can with perfect form (targets quadriceps, core).

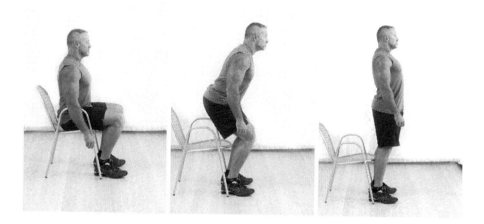

Squat with Arms in Front

Stand with legs shoulder width apart beside a chair or bar if you need it for support. Slowly sit back on your heels into a squat. Keep your knees in line with your toes (don't let your knees knock together). Pause and then squeeze your butt cheeks together as you stand. As you get stronger, pause in the knee-bent position for a count of 2 and then 4 for added strengthening (targets quadriceps, hamstrings, and glutes).

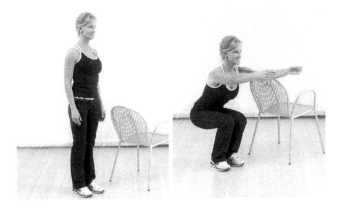

Fitness Ball Single-Leg Squat

Stand facing away from a fitness ball, about 2 feet in front of it. Place your right foot on the ball. With your weight on your left leg, bend your left knee and let your right leg roll back on the ball. Keep your left knee straight over your toes. Pause and return to a stand. Build to 12–15 repetitions with each leg. When this gets easy, hold 3 or 5 lb. dumbbells in your hands (targets quads and glutes, balance).

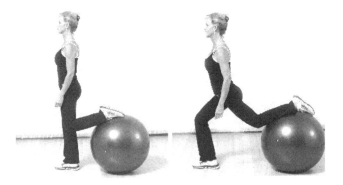

Sumo Squat

Stand with your feet more than shoulder width apart and toes pointed out to the sides at a 45-degree angle. Hold a 3–5 lb. dumbbell with both hands, and let your arms hang straight down. Slowly bend your knees, all the while keeping your knees out over your toes. Use weights that let you easily do 15 reps while maintaining perfect form (targets glutes, quads, and inner thighs).

For added difficulty, hold a 10 lb. dumbbell in both hands between your legs.

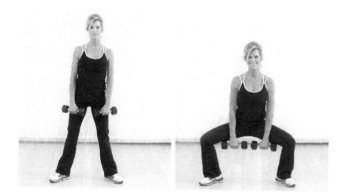

LEGS–HAMSTRINGS

Pick one of these exercises to start with. Change every 4–6 weeks.

Hip Bridge

Lying on your back with heels tucked close to your buttocks, lift your buttocks off the ground so your body forms a straight line from knees to shoulders. Hold for 2 seconds, then slowly lower over a 2-second count. Do 8–12 reps (targets hamstrings, glutes, and low back).

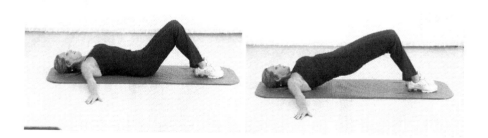

For added difficulty, straighten your right leg from the knee and do the movement using only the left leg to lift your body. Keep the right leg straight during the exercise. Do 8–12 reps on each side.

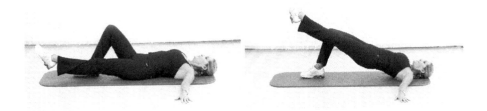

For even more difficulty, straighten your right leg with your toes pointing at the ceiling. Keep your leg pointed toward the ceiling as you raise your body with your left leg. Do 8–12 reps, then repeat with the left leg straight.

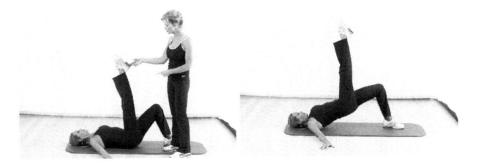

Dumbbell Leg Curl

Lie facedown on a bench and have your workout partner place a light dumbbell between your feet, with one end of the dumbbell resting on the soles of your shoes. Bend your knees and bring your feet toward your buttocks. Hold the dumbbell tight between your feet. Keep your hips flat on the bench. Pause and then lower the weight to the starting position. Do 8–10 reps (targets hamstrings and glutes).

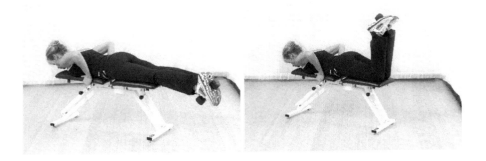

Hamstring Ball Roll

Lie on your back with your legs straight and your calves resting on a stability ball. You are in a straight line from your shoulders to your heels. Bend your knees and roll the ball toward your buttocks. Keep your hips elevated, and you will feel your hamstrings and buttocks working as you bring the stability ball as close to your buttocks as you can. Just your heels should be resting on the ball at this time. It is easiest to do this exercise with your arms extended out to the side on the floor for balance. Do as many as you can with your goal being 3 sets of 8–12 repetitions. For added difficulty and better core strengthening, keep your arms at your sides (targets hamstrings, low back, and glutes).

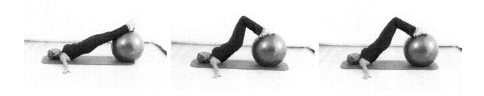

LEGS–CALVES

Pick one of these exercises to start with. Change every 4–6 weeks. Remember the balance exercises will also strengthen your legs and especially your calves.

Seated Calf Raise

Sit with 5 or 10 lb. dumbbells resting on each knee. Slowly lift your knees and come up on the balls of your feet. Pause for a count of 2 and then slowly lower. Make sure that you're using your calves to raise the weights and not your arms. Repeat 12–15 times (targets calves).

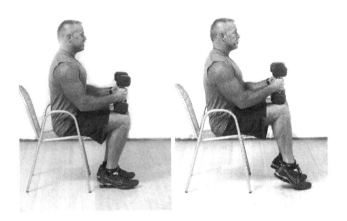

Standing Calf Raise

Stand on a step or a block with the toes and ball of your right foot at the edge of the step. Hold on to a wall or chair with your left hand for balance. Cross your left foot behind your right ankle and balance yourself on the ball of your right foot. Lower your heel as far as you can till you feel a stretch in the back of your calf. Lift your heel as high as you can, pause, and return to the starting position. Do 10–15 reps and repeat with the left leg (targets calves, balance).

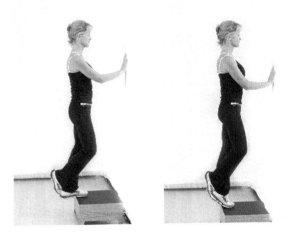

BALANCE

Pick one of these exercises to start with. Change every 4–6 weeks.

Eyes Closed

Stand on a thick folded towel with your feet shoulder width apart. Stand tall with your abdominal muscles engaged (say *sshhh* to engage them). Close your eyes and visualize the upright position.

Balance on One Leg

Stand with your hand on a chair or bar for support. Shift your weight to your left leg and lift the right leg off the floor. Try letting go of your support or only resting your fingertips on the bar for balance. Your goal is to stand on one leg for 30 seconds. Turn around and repeat it standing on your right leg.

Advanced

Fold a bath towel several times over, place it on the floor, and stand on the center of the towel. This will give you a slightly unstable surface because the towel is soft.

Advanced

Try doing the one-leg balance with your eyes shut. Keep the chair back close so you can steady yourself as needed.

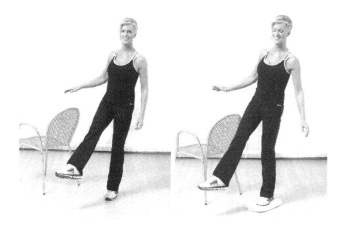

Toe-Stand Balance

Stand facing a sturdy chair or bar with your hands resting lightly on it. Rise up onto your toes and try to let go of the chair and balance for a count of 10. When you are an expert, raise up on your toes and, still holding on gently, shift your weight to the right leg and try to balance on your toes on one leg. You will feel the muscles of your entire leg and your core engage. Keep your head high and stomach strong (say *sshhh*).

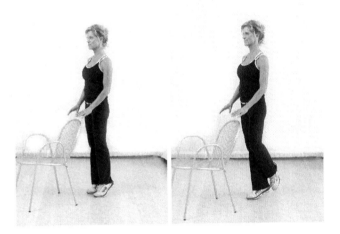

Advanced One-Leg Balance

Stand next to a chair or bar with your right arm resting on it. Slowly lift your left leg behind you. Let your body tilt forward so that you maintain a straight line from the tip of your head to your toes. This will mean that you have to engage your back and stomach muscles to hold your position firm. Bend forward till you are at a 45-degree angle and balance there for 10 seconds. Then if you have the flexibility, continue to tip your body forward until you are looking at the ground and your left leg is extended straight behind you. Balance there for 10 seconds, then slowly return to a stand. Repeat on the right. Work up so you can do 10 on each side without holding on for balance.

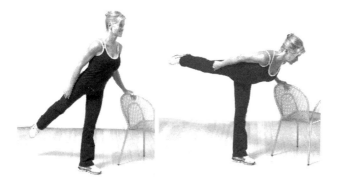

One-Leg Balance with Twist

Balance on your left leg with your right leg bent in front of you and your hands on your hips. As you move your right leg behind you, reach your right arm across your body. Your goal is to try to touch the floor on the outside of your left foot. Do all while balancing on your left leg, and keep your right foot from touching the floor. Return to your starting position and repeat 5 times (if you can) and then switch legs (targets thighs, glutes, hamstrings, core, and balance).

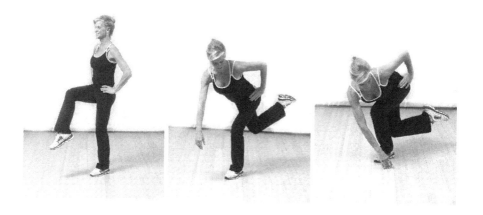

CORE

Although you'll see everyone in the gym dropping to do 50 sit-ups, they are defeating the purpose on several fronts. The first problem is the number 50. Any exercise you do where you can do more than 20 is not building strength efficiently. Your best bet is to slow down the exercise so you recruit more muscle fibers and build strength efficiently. Doing 50 sit-ups does not provide enough muscle resistance to build strength. Working your abs slowly will recruit the maximal number of muscle fibers and provide optimal strength gains. Find 1 or 2 exercises that are hard enough that you can only do 8–15 reps.

The second problem is with the word *sit-up*. It's a bad choice of an exercise to build core strength. You see, any exercise where you raise your body up from the floor is using your hip flexor muscles far more than it uses your abdominal muscles. So with the classic sit-up, you are training your hip flexors but not your abdominal/core muscles. The sit-up is not only ineffective, but it is also potentially dangerous. It can easily strain your low back, a situation we want to avoid. The exercises that follow are safe for your back and will develop all four of your abdominal muscles, providing the strong core you need. Your core muscles include your rectus abdominis muscle, which is your six-pack. But there are three other sets of muscles that run underneath the rectus muscles. These three sets of muscles run diagonally and across your belly and are the ones we want to strengthen. The following exercises focus on strengthening these. Core also includes your low back muscles. They work in tandem with your abdominal muscles to provide support for your back. Pick a combination of exercises from the list below that work both.

You should do 2–3 of the following exercises as part of your weight training program. After 4–6 weeks, switch exercises.

Resistance One-Leg Crunch

Lie on your back with your knees bent with your feet on the floor. Lift your right knee and resist the movement with your right arm. Hold for a count of 2 and then return to the starting position. Repeat on the left. That is 1 repetition. Work up so you can do 8–12 reps (targets abs).

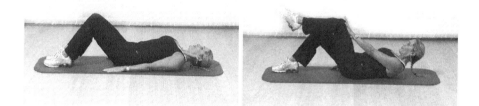

My Crunch

Lie on the floor; with fingers lightly behind your ears, slowly raise your shoulders and buttocks at the same time. If you are doing the exercise correctly, then you will feel your lower abdominal muscles along with your six-pack engage. It is more important to try to lift your buttocks off the floor than lift your shoulders. Hold for 2 seconds and slowly return to your starting position. Do as many as you can (targets abs).

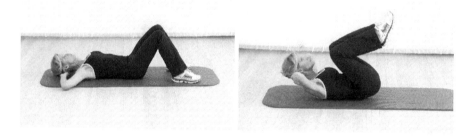

Suitcase Walk

Hold a 3 or 5 lb. dumbbell in your right hand at your side. Keeping your body in perfect alignment, walk as far as you can without discomfort. Repeat with the dumbbell in the other hand. Walk progressively longer distances to challenge your core. Stand tall with stomach strong and shoulders back. Remember to check yourself by saying *sshhh*. This will engage your core the correct way. Increase the amount of weight you carry as the exercise gets easier (targets core-stabilizing muscles).

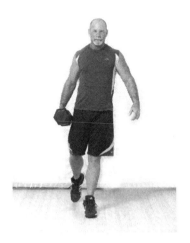

Fitness Ball Crunch

Lie on a fitness ball that is the right size for you. The correct-size ball is one that when you sit on it, your knees are bent at a right angle. Lie back on the ball so your thighs and torso are parallel to the floor. Cross your arms over your chest. In a slow, controlled manner, contract your stomach, lifting your shoulders off the ball, and gently tuck your chin to your chest. As you raise your shoulders, slowly exhale. Rise no more than 45 degrees. Then slowly return to your starting position. Inhale as you lower. The closer your feet are together, the harder the exercise. For beginners, place your shoulders and upper back on the ball with your thighs and torso parallel to the floor. Do crunches with the stability ball supporting your entire torso. As that gets easy, place the ball farther down your back so that more of your upper body is off the ball. You will find this is a much harder way to do the crunch (targets abs).

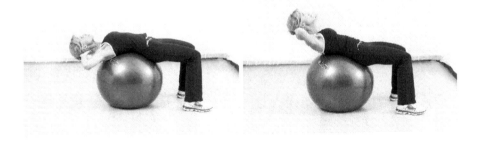

Plank

This is one of my favorite core-strengthening exercises.

Assume a modified push-up position with your forearms resting on the floor. Elbows should be under your shoulders and bent at 90 degrees. Keep your torso steady and your body in a straight line from your head to your toes. Do not let your stomach sag. Hold for as long as you can. Your goal is to hold this for 30 seconds (targets core-stabilizing muscles).

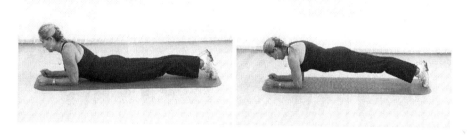

Single-Leg Lowering

Lie on your back with both legs straight up in the air (never lock your knees). Press the small of your back into the floor. It is best to place your hands slightly under the small of your back to make sure it never arches up. Point your foot and slowly lower your right leg as far as you can while maintaining perfect form. Your goal is to lower it 2–3 inches from the floor. Bring your right leg back up and repeat with the left. Do 8–12 reps (targets abs, quads).

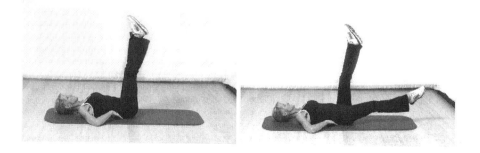

Dryland Swimming

Lie on your stomach on an exercise pad (you might want a towel under your hips for comfort) with your arms extended overhead. Lift your arms and legs off the floor at the same time so they are about 6–8 inches off the ground. Keep looking at the floor. Kick your legs up and down like you are swimming. While you are kicking, move your arms from above your head to your sides and back over your head. Kick for as long as you can, avoiding soreness in your low back (targets back, glutes, and legs).

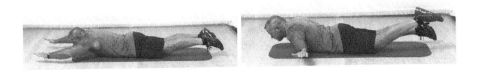

Cable (or Dumbbell) Woodchopper

Stand with your right side toward the weight stack of a cable machine. Grab the rope handle of a high pulley with both hands. Pull the cable across your body until your hands are across your body just outside your left knee. Slowly reverse the move to return to the starting position. Do 12–15 reps (targets abs, shoulders, back, and legs).

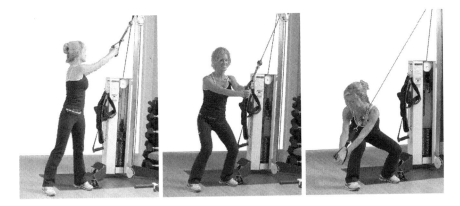

To Use Dumbbells

Hold light dumbbell with hand over handgrip with your arms extended above your right shoulder. Keep your arms straight, but don't lock your elbows. Bend your knees and lower the weight down and across your body until your hands reach the outside of your left ankle. Pause then quickly reverse the movement, pausing at the top. That is 1 repetition. Use a weight that is light enough that you can do 12–15 repetitions.

Reverse Cable Woodchopper

Now attach the rope handle to the low pulley cable. Bend over and grab the rope with both hands. Your arms should be nearly straight and just outside your right knee. Keeping your arms straight, pull the rope up across your body until your hands are in line with your left ear. Slowly reverse the movement and return to your original position in a controlled manner. Do 12–15 reps (targets abdominals, shoulders, back, and legs).

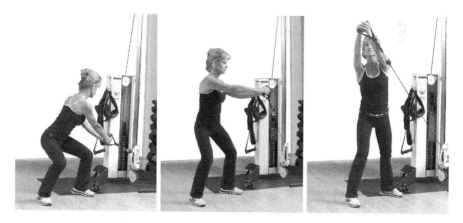

To Use Dumbbells

Crouch down using a light dumbbell with hand over handgrip with your arms extended beside your right bent knee. Keep your arms straight but don't lock your elbows. Straighten your knees as you lift the weight across your body until your hands are raised over your head past your left shoulder. Pause then slowly lower the weight back to the starting position. That is 1 repetition. Use a weight that is light enough that you can do 15–20 repetitions on each side.

BACK

This section supplements the lower back work found in the core section with more focused upper back work. This should be one of your target spots as we fight the inevitable dowager's hump as our shoulders slump with old age. You can combat the humped posture with a strong back and a balance between chest and upper back strength. In other words, don't overdo your chest work just because it is an area you can see and admire.

Wall Slide

Stand with your buttocks, upper back, and head against the wall. Raise your arms over your head so your shoulders, elbows, and wrists also touch the wall. Maintaining these points of contact, bend your arms until your elbows are tucked in at your sides. You should feel a contraction in your shoulders and the muscles between your shoulder blades. Reverse the move. Do 10 repetitions (targets upper back).

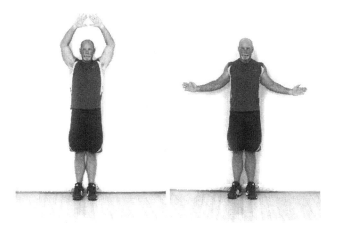

Fitness Ball Y

Lie on a fitness ball with your legs straight and your chest off the ball. Let your fists rest on the floor with your arms hanging down in front of your shoulders. Lift your arms up and to the sides, forming at 45-degree angles to form a Y. While you raise your arms, focus on moving your shoulder blades back and down. Reverse the move back to the starting position. When you can repeat this 8–10 times, then do it holding 1–3 lb. weights (targets back).

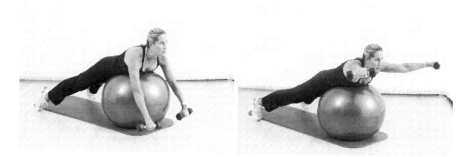

Fitness Ball T

Lie on a fitness ball with your legs straight and your chest off the ball. Let your hands rest on the floor with your arms straight. Squeeze your shoulder blades together and raise your arms straight out to the sides, forming a T with your torso and arms. Reverse the move back to the starting position. When you can repeat this 8–10 times, then do it holding 1–3 lb. weights (targets back).

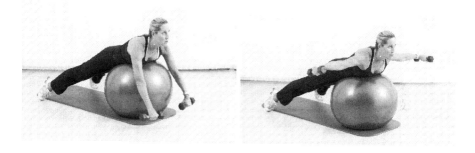

Dumbbell Single-Arm Row

Holding a dumbbell in your right hand, place your left knee and left hand on a bench. Your right arm should be straight and hang just in front of your shoulder. Keeping your back flat and right elbow close to your body, pull the dumbbell up and back toward your hip. Pause and then slowly lower the weight. Repeat 8 times, then switch sides (targets upper back).

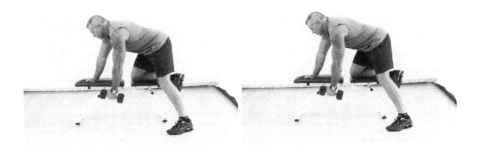

Lat Pull Down

Sit at the lat pull-down station. Adjust the leg pads so your legs fit secure underneath. Grab the bar and begin by pulling your shoulder blades down and together. Keep them pinched tight and then pull the bar down toward the floor (or, if you are using a bar, then pull it down to chest height). Keep your back straight and move slowly through the full range of motion. Do 12–15 reps (targets back).

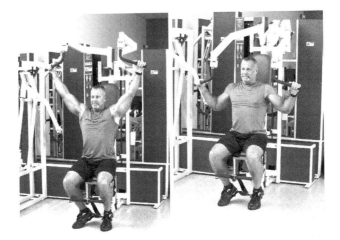

CHEST

Select one exercise from this section and change exercises every 4–6 weeks.

Wall Push-ups (the perfect beginner's exercise)

Stand at arm's length from the wall. Put both hands on the wall at chest level. Slowly bend your elbows to the count of 4 and then slowly straighten them. Repeat 12 times. When this is easy, go to the modified push-up below (targets chest).

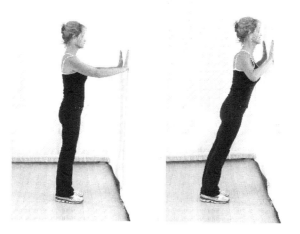

Push-ups on Knees

I know these are girl push-ups, but done correctly, they will result in impressive improvements in your strength. Once you can do 12 of these with perfect form, then it is time to do them in the regular push-up position. Keep your core strong throughout the push-up by maintaining a straight line from your knees to the top of your head.

Kneel on the floor with your knees on a pad. Walk your arms out until your body is in a straight line with your knees bent. In this modified push-up position, I want you to slowly lower your body (keeping a straight line from the tip of your head to your knees) until you are barely touching the floor and then slowly return to the starting position, keeping perfect form (targets chest).

Do 6–12 reps in each of the three-hand positions illustrated.

A) Normal push-up position—elbows are at a 90-degree angle with your hands right under your elbows.

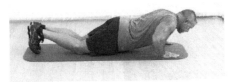

B) Wide-arm position—hands are placed out past your elbows so the angle of your elbows is about 120 degrees.

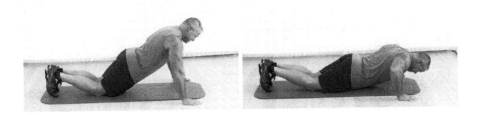

C) Diamond—place your hands so that your thumb and index fingers touch each other and make the shape of a diamond.

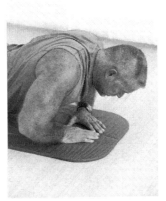

Alternating Dumbbell Press on a Fitness Ball

Lie on a fitness ball with your upper back resting on the ball. Bend your knees, place your feet on the floor, and keep your body in a straight line throughout the exercise. Hold a 5 lb. dumbbell in each hand with your elbows bent and the dumbbell at chest level. Alternating arms, press the dumbbell to the ceiling. As you lower the right arm in a controlled manner, raise the dumbbell in your left arm to the ceiling. Keep your core strong. The closer your feet are together, the more you will work your core. Do 12–20 reps (targets chest, abs).

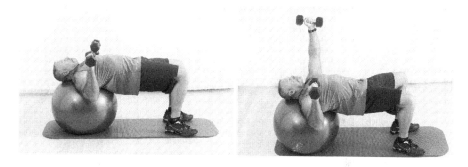

Dumbbell Incline Fly

Lie faceup on an incline bench. Hold 3–5 lb. dumbbells straight over your chest with your palms facing each other. Slowly open your arms, keeping your hands in line with your shoulders. Stop when the weights are level with your chest. Pause and return to the starting position. Repeat 12–20 times (targets chest).

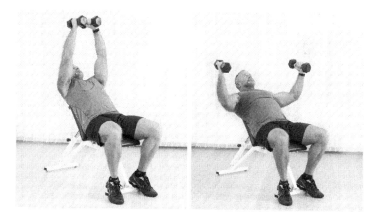

SHOULDERS

Select one exercise from this section and change exercises every 4–6 weeks.

Shoulder Shrug

Stand holding a 3–5 lb. dumbbell in each hand, palms facing toward each other. Shrug your shoulders up to your ears and pause. Slowly lower your shoulders. Repeat 12 times (targets shoulders).

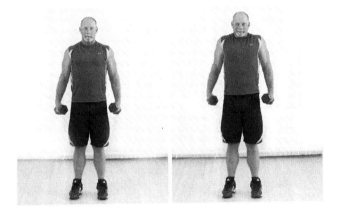

Dumbbell Upright Row

Stand holding a pair of dumbbells in front of your thighs, arms straight and palms facing your body. Lift your upper arms and bring the dumbbells up until your hands are just below your chin. Pause and then lower the weight back to the starting position. Do 12–15 reps (targets shoulders).

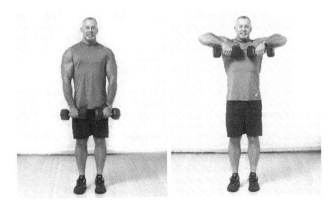

Controlled Fly

Kneel on a bench with your right leg and right arm on the bench. In your left hand, you are holding a 1 or 3 lb. weight with the palm facing you. Keep your back flat and stomach strong during the exercise. Slowly lift the weight out to the side till your arm is parallel to the floor. Repeat 10 times with each arm (targets shoulders).

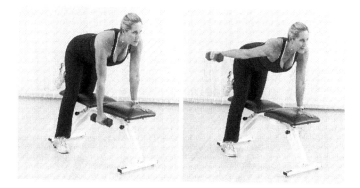

Toss and Catch

Play toss and catch with a beach ball or light medicine ball. As the exercise gets easier, you can increase the weight of the ball. Keep your stomach engaged (tense the muscles like you're going to be punched in the stomach) throughout your game, especially right before you throw the ball (targets shoulders and abs).

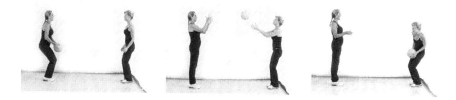

Internal/External Rotation

This is a great one to stabilize your shoulder girdle and prevent injuries.

Stand with your arm at your side, a 1–3 lb. dumbbell in your hand. Bend your elbow at 90 degrees so your forearm and hand point forward with your palm facing toward your body. Slowly bring your arm across your body until your hand touches your abdomen. Return to the starting position. Keep your elbow in a fixed position so your shoulder rotator cuff muscles do all the work. Then repeat the exercise so that your hands rotate away from your body and face out in either direction. Again, keep your elbows at a 90-degree angle and fixed in position. Do 12–15 reps of the full exercise (targets shoulders, internal and external rotators).

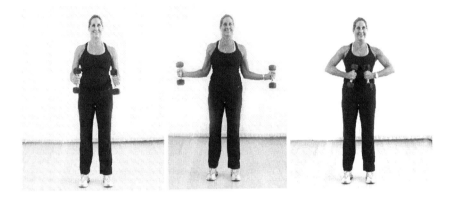

Alternating Shoulder Dumbbell Press

By alternating your arms, you also get core strengthening with the exercise.

Sit with your back supported. Engage your core (like you are preparing to be punched). This will provide a solid core to protect your back and double the value of the exercise by working your stomach muscles. Hold a 1–3 lb. dumbbell in each hand at shoulder level with palms facing each other. Press the dumbbell in your right hand straight above you until your arm is straight and the weight is above your head. Then slowly lower the weight to the starting position. Repeat on the left. Do a total of 8–12 per side (targets shoulders and core).

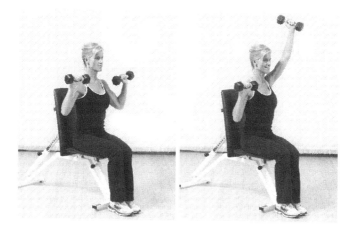

Advanced

Do the same exercise standing or stand on one leg to challenge your core. Keep your abdominal muscles engaged.

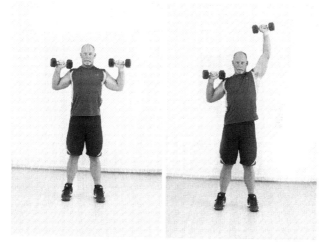

Lateral Raises 3 Ways

This is one of my favorite exercises and part of my exercise routine. To use all three heads of the deltoid, you will do the standard lateral raise using three different hand positions. Do this exercise with low weight and slow, controlled movements.

Stand tall, stomach firm, holding a 1, 3, or 5 lb. dumbbell in each hand. With your hands facing forward and arms straight, slowly raise both dumbbells at a 45-degree angle to shoulder level. Your thumbs should be pointing at the ceiling. Do not raise them above shoulder level. Slowly lower to the count of 2 or 4. You will feel this primarily in the anterior head of the deltoid (your shoulder muscle).

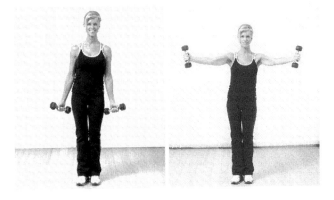

Next, turn your hands to face each other and lift the dumbbells slowly to the side. All your knuckles will be directed toward the ceiling. Do not raise them above shoulder level. This will strengthen the middle head of the deltoid. Slowly lower.

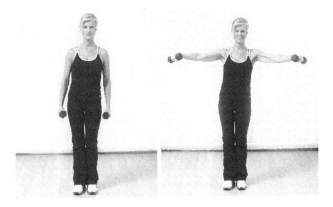

Lastly, turn your hands facing the back with your pinkies on top. Slowly lift to the side, again stopping at shoulder height. You will feel this engage the posterior head of the deltoid. Slowly lower. Repeat the entire set (all three moves are 1 set) 8 times.

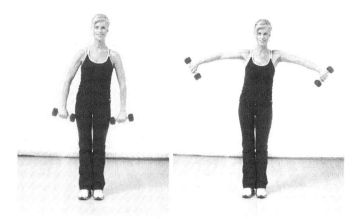

COOLDOWN (5-10 minutes after every exercise session)

The cooldown is important to minimize muscle soreness and fatigue. During exercise, your body accumulates lactic acid (a by-product of muscle work). We associate lactic acid buildup with muscle soreness. The cooldown period gives your body a chance to clear the lactic acid from your muscles and so minimizes postworkout discomfort.

Walk slowly for about 10 minutes after you finish exercising to gently return your heart rate to its resting level. Or you can simply do a slower version of whatever exercise you were doing. Continue walking until you are breathing normally and can easily carry on a conversation. During your cooldown period is the best time to stretch. But wait until your heart rate has slowed and is approaching your resting rate.

Do not stop exercising abruptly. If you simply stop after exercising vigorously, then there is a good chance your blood pressure will drop and you will get light-headed and dizzy. Keep moving. It's what all the experts say and for very good reason. Especially if you have any history of coronary artery disease, you need to make the cooldown period an important priority. Think of the cooldown period as "active rest," where you are gently returning your body to its pre-exercise state.

And don't forget rehydrating. Unless you have been exercising at a high intensity for an hour or more, water is the best fluid for rehydration. None of us need the calories of the electrolyte drinks, and rarely do we lose enough salt with routine exercise to require extra salt found in these sport drinks.

GENERAL STRETCHES FOR YOUR COOLDOWN

Maintaining flexibility of your muscles will increase your range of motion and provide agility. It is also important to minimize injury. The most important and permanent way to increase your flexibility is to do every exercise you do through the full range of movement. Exercises like lunges, squats, and even push-ups should be done by moving your body through its full pain-free range of motion. As you move your body as far as it can, make sure you keep good form during every repetition. But because they feel so good, I have included my favorite static stretches. When you do the static stretches, start slowly, breathe deeply, and push just to the limit of pain. You will find that as your joint warms up, you will be able to go a little farther each time. Use your breath to help you relax into each stretch. Take a slow, deep breath in through your nose and then relax into the stretch as you exhale through your mouth. Think about your breath and consciously breathe deep in through your nose, filling your lungs down to their bases. This will help you relax and make the most of each stretch. Bouncing or forcing the stretch is actually counterproductive. *Do not bounce.* Plan to do the majority of your stretching program while you are cooling down, while your muscles are still warm from exercising.

Kneeling Quad Stretch

Kneel with your right leg bent in front of you with your knee at a 90-degree angle and your left knee on a mat for cushioning. Keep your body vertical and gently press your hips forward to feel a stretch in the front of the left thigh and hip. Hold for a count of 10, then relax. Repeat 5–10 times and then repeat on the other side.

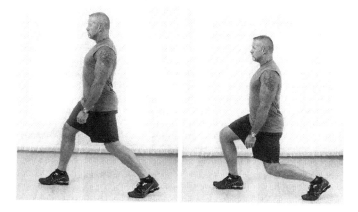

Quadriceps Standing Stretch

Stand facing a chair, holding on to the back lightly for balance. Bend the right knee and grab your ankle with your right hand. Hold for a count of 5, exhaling during the stretch. Try to balance by lifting your hands off the back of the chair on during the stretch to engage core strengthening.

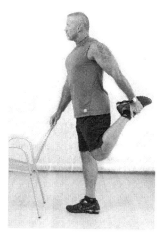

Piriformis Stretch

Lying on your back, bend your right knee with your knee at a 90-degree angle and your foot on the floor. Rest your left ankle on your right leg and let your knee relax out to the side. Gently pull your right knee to your chest and feel the stretch in the left buttock. Hold for a count of 5, exhaling during the stretch.

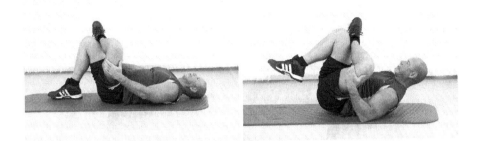

Lying Hamstring Stretch

Lie on your back with both legs straight on the floor and arms by your sides. Bring your right knee to your chest. Place both hands behind your right knee and slowly straighten your right leg. It is OK if you need to lower your right leg to get your knee straight. Hold the straight-leg position for a count of 5, slowly exhaling while you straighten it. Bend the knee again and repeat the exercise 5–10 times on each side.

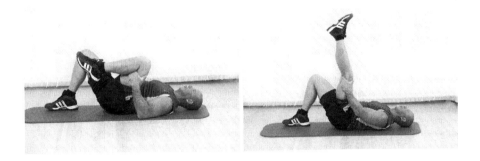

Calf Stretch

Stand on a bottom stair, holding on to the railing for support. Edge your feet back so your heels are off the step. Slowly rise up on your toes and hold for a count of 2. Then lower your body, keeping your knees straight until your heels are below the step and you feel a stretch up the back of your leg.

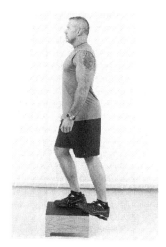

The Cat

Kneel on all fours. Slowly round your back, tucking your head and bringing your shoulders as close as you can to your hips. Pause for the count of 2 and return to the starting position. Then slowly arch your back. Pause and return to the neutral starting position. That is 1 repetition. Do 10 repetitions.

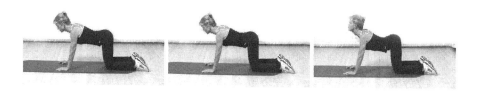

Trunk Twister

Lie on your back on the floor with your arms extended out at shoulder level. Raise your right leg until your toes point to the ceiling. Keeping your leg straight and your shoulders glued to the floor, slowly lower your leg across your body until your toe touches the floor on the left side of your body. Pause at the point that your shoulder wants to lift off the floor. Raise your leg back up in the air and then lower it to the floor. Repeat with your left leg. Do 5–10 repetitions on each side.

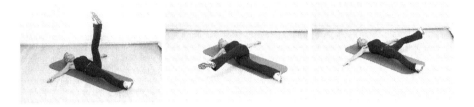

Hamstrings

Lie on your back with your arms out to the side. Raise your right leg into the air. Keeping your knee straight, point and flex your foot 8 times. This will provide a nice stretch for your hamstrings while keeping your back safe. Repeat on the left.

For an extra stretch, grab on to the back of your thigh and gently pull your leg toward you. Breathe in and hold for a count of 2 as you exhale.

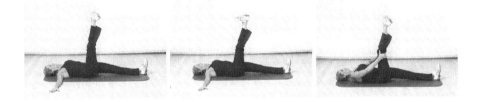

Floor Chest Stretch

Lie faceup on a foam roll with your head supported. Extend your arms out to your sides with your palms facing the ceiling. You will feel a stretch across your chest. Take slow, easy breaths and hold the stretch for 30 seconds. Repeat 3 times.

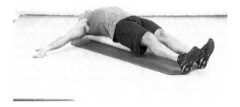

Supine Tuck and Curl

Lie flat on your back, knees bent and feet on the floor. Moving slowly, tilt your pelvis and lift your hips off the floor slightly, then lower. Do 6 reps.

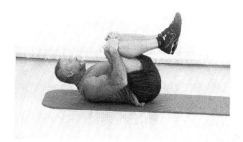

Knee-to-Chest Pose

Lie on your back with your legs fully extended. Draw one knee to your chest and hold it with both hands. Breathe in and, as you breathe out, pull your knee to your chest. Hold for 3–5 breaths. Switch legs and repeat.

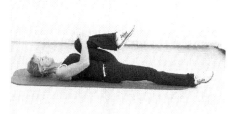

Side Stretch

Stand with your feet apart and stretch your arms over your head as you inhale. Draw a big circle with the fingertips of your right hand as you exhale through your mouth and reach to the side. Hold for a count of two and as you inhale and return to the upright position. Exhale and lower your arms to your sides. Repeat for a total of 8 on each side. This is a very relaxing way to finish your exercise session.

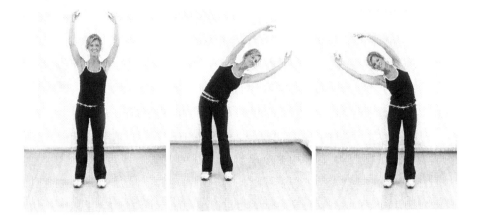

I believe the wise men who say that we are masters of our own fate. Our life is ours, our health is ours, our happiness is ours. Once you take responsibility for your health, you have the power to change it. Stop blaming, stop complaining, and slowly, with love and tenderness, pick yourself up off the couch and go for your first walk. It is the walk of your lifetime.

Exercise to Treat Low Back Pain

It hurts to move. It hurts to bend or walk; maybe it hurts to reach. So you stop doing the things that hurt. Right? You figure the pain you're feeling must be a signal to stop because you're damaging something. Right? So you stop moving, and you subtly alter how you walk, bend, and reach so it doesn't hurt. But instead of feeling better, you're not. In fact, you're hurting more. How can that be? You've stopped doing the painful stuff. You should be getting better. Right? Wrong. Wrong. Wrong. Wrong.

Low back pain is one of the most common health-related problems in the world. Despite its prevalence, we are at the very early stages of our understanding of how to treat or cure chronic pain. Pain management is a relatively new board-certified medical specialty, and we are in our infancy of understanding. However, there are things we do know. We know that you are in control of your health. Funny, I'm pretty sure I say that in every chapter of this book. And I also keep saying that you are the only one in control of your disease. Is it sinking in yet? Like all the other diseases in this book, the best way to treat low back pain is with regular exercise and activity. You see, the only proven treatment of many pain diseases is regular exercise, an anti-inflammatory diet, and maintaining your optimal weight. There are no miracle pills or injections or surgeries. They can all help, but if you don't take responsibility for your disease and take the reins in its treatment, then our medical approaches don't stand a chance.

Doctors know how important exercise is to control chronic pain. They tell every one of their patients to get exercising. But although doctors know a lot about your disease, we don't have a quick, easy answer to your question "So how do I start?" or "What do I do?" Well, here you go. Here is your start. The following is a guided program to start you on a safe and effective program to change your life and treat your disease.

I know pain. I spend my days caring for patients with chronic pain. But I also know pain because I have been living with low back pain for 30 years. I have watched from a personal vantage point as the medical profession floundered to explain or even control my pain, all with little success. Now I have found ways to live despite my pain. And with medical knowledge behind me, I hope to save you my trial and error of my experience. I now understand that low back pain is a disease. It is a disease that if you give into it, then it will win. So I'm here to help you fight the fight.

ACUTE AND CHRONIC PAIN

There are two types of pain: acute and chronic. Acute pain, by definition, is a pain that has been present for less than 6 weeks, and it often resolves on its own. But recurrence rates are upward of 50%, so although it may resolve quickly, the chances of it returning are high. Maintaining a high level of physical conditioning and core strength can minimize the chance of repeated pain flares. The exercises at the end of this chapter are as important for you as for the chronic pain patient. You must focus on strengthening the weakened area to prevent recurrent injuries and also on aerobic conditioning. If low back pain is your problem, then focus on core strengthening. If recurrent ankle strains are your problem, then strengthen those weak ankles. Physical therapists are excellent for this, but you must have one that teaches you the active strengthening exercises you need to learn. Stretching and massage feel good, but they are not the most effective treatments for pain. You need active exercise to combat and prevent your acute pain flares. So remember, your acute pain will likely become chronic if you don't get moving.

Acute nonspecific low back pain is usually due to musculoskeletal factors and will resolve on its own, if you don't baby it. If you have symptoms of ongoing neurological damage such as weakness in your legs or loss of bowel or bladder control, then seek medical treatment quickly. And please see your doctor for cardiac clearance before starting your exercise program.

This is what we know about exercise for acute back pain:

1. Continue your usual daily activity as soon as possible. You must limit bed rest to only 1–2 days, and then you have got to get moving.
2. A low-stress aerobic exercise program can help prevent debilitation from inactivity. These programs include walking, biking, swimming.
3. You can start your low-stress activity program usually during the first 2 weeks after an injury.
4. Add in conditioning exercises for trunk/core muscles as your pain resolves.
5. Stretching exercises for back muscles provide little benefit. They are specifically not recommended as the sole treatment for back pain.

These 5 steps will jump-start you on your way to easing your acute pain flare, but they will also help prevent further recurrences of your pain. If you stick with it, that is. So what specific exercises should you do for acute back pain? The same types of exercise we recommend for chronic back pain. The exercises at the end of the chapter focus on trunk strength and mobility. Pick several to start with. Master your form and then add other exercises from the list to provide variety and continually challenge your muscles.

The second type of low back pain is chronic low back pain. By definition, it has lasted longer than 3 months. It is one of the most complex diseases known. It can start slowly or suddenly; it can result from major trauma or be the result of undetectable repeated episodes of microtrauma that occur over time. Chronic pain is a disease, and the worst thing you can do for this disease is to stop moving. Chronic pain thrives on inactivity and the weakened muscles that result when you baby your pain.

There is an important distinction between these two types of pain. Acute pain serves as a warning signal for the body, a signal of impending damage to the painful area. We react to acute pain appropriately by guarding and immobilizing the injured body part. An easy-to-understand example of acute pain is the pain of a broken arm or sprained ankle. Treatment of acute pain is immobilization or bed rest for 1–2 days but then a return slowly to regular activity. We used to recommend bed rest for weeks after a flare of acute low back pain, but no longer. The important take-home point is that even with acute pain, rest should only be for 1–2 days. Bed rest and inactivity are your enemies. Your doctor will encourage you to walk around the house and do whatever you can tolerate to keep the ravages of bed rest and muscle wasting from compounding your pain problems. Prolonged bed rest is almost a guarantee that your acute pain will escalate into a chronic pain disease. "Move it or lose it" is your mantra.

On the other hand, chronic low back pain is a disease like hypertension or diabetes. It is a disease of the nervous system pain pathways. It is not a signal of tissue damage. It is not a signal to stop moving and baby your pain. Instead, your pain results from diseased nerve pathways that have run amok and are sending pain signals unrelated to tissue injury or damage. So just because it hurts to move doesn't mean you are doing damage. You're not. We know that. But you should always check with your doctor if you're concerned. Many of my chronic pain patients suffer an occasional severe flare of their pain. And when I am concerned or it seems extra severe, I will evaluate with an MRI. But the vast majority of times, there is absolutely no change in the MRI. In other words, there is no new disc protrusion and no worsening of the disc bulges that are present. There is nothing changed in their spine to explain their worsened pain. It is just those darn nerves screaming louder to be heard. And most often there was nothing that they did or didn't do to cause the pain. Those diseased pathways just start screaming. I use the example of a fire alarm to explain this to my patients. A fire alarm starts to ring to signal a fire. The firemen race to the scene and put out the fire. No more fire. But the fire alarm keeps ringing. It keeps ringing and ringing and ringing. The fire was extinguished weeks ago, maybe months or years ago, but the fire alarm is still ringing. Is there a fire? No. Instead, there is a short circuit in the fire alarm. It is ringing without any reason. It is not signaling a fire. It's just ringing out of control. And that is what chronic pain is. There is a short circuit in your nervous system and your pain pathways are ringing off the wall, but they are not signaling any real damage. The damage was done months or years ago, and it has long since healed. What you are left with is a short circuit in your pain pathways. The pain is no longer related to an injury. The injury is in the nerve pathways themselves.

WHY EXERCISE?

Our natural response to pain, whether it is acute or chronic, is the same. We stop doing what hurts. And that means we stop moving or move in ways that protect the painful area. As you decrease your activity level in a futile attempt to control your pain, your muscles weaken very quickly. And your weakened muscles add to your pain; they spasm and cramp and are no longer able to support your aching spine. So as the chronic pain patient becomes less active, his pain worsens. Instead of healing, your inactivity is making your disease much worse. We naturally think that if walking hurts or exercising hurts, then we shouldn't do it. But with chronic pain disease, pain is not a signal of tissue damage. It serves no function. It just hurts. By the time a patient with chronic pain is seen by a pain specialist, up to 80% of their pain is due to muscle wasting and weakness that no amount of medicine can combat.

The only thing to break the spiral and begin to cure the disease is activity and exercise. The rest of what medicine has to offer are temporary fixes or Band-Aids for the problem. Just like we manage diabetes and hypertension with pills, so do we control pain with a mixture of medications, pain injections, and surgery. When your nervous system is diseased and your pain runs rampant, even the best surgery done by the most perfect surgeon cannot cure the disease. At this point, the disease is in the nervous system itself, and even though the perfect surgeon fixes the herniated disc, the pain pathways are damaged and continue to send pain signals out of control. Surgery fails often enough that it has its own name—failed back syndrome. This is an actual medical diagnosis, and that is a shame. Not because the surgeons are bad, but because we still know so little about how to effectively treat this terrible disease.

However, there are things you can do. I know. I've taken control of my chronic back pain, and I will share with you what I have learned from 30 years of my own trial and error, combined with the latest scientific information available in medicine. Only you can cure yourself. As a pain management specialist, the reason I prescribe pills or do injections is to provide temporary pain relief so each patient can get active and heal himself or herself. The right type of exercise will reeducate your pain pathways to function normally.

SAFETY PRECAUTIONS

With all this cheerleading to get you moving, there are caveats:

1. Be aware of the danger signs of neurologic damage. Most flares of pain, although scary, don't signal a worsening of your disease. But there are some signs that concern doctors and should be evaluated quickly. If you are experiencing new acute pain that runs down your leg or if the pain is associated with new numbness, weakness, tingling or loss of bowel or bladder function, then do not treat yourself. Stop exercise and get evaluated by your doctor soon. Exercise is indicated for the majority of low back pain problems, but only your doctor can decide if it is the appropriate treatment for you.

2. Go slow, go smart. Even though your pain is a disease and has become dissociated from its normal warning function, that doesn't mean you should disregard it entirely. You must learn to listen to your body and allow that mild pain is often fine, but you should never push yourself too hard. If you push too hard, then you will experience a severe pain flare, and I doubt you will give this book another try. Baby steps for you.

Because of the nature of your disease, this chapter is different from the others. Your exercise focus is on movement, not exercise per se. If you have minimal pain and want a more aggressive program, then I refer you to the high blood pressure chapter for a more intensive exercise program.

LET'S GET STARTED: YOUR EXERCISE PROGRAM

For the rest of this chapter, I am going to use the term *physical activity* rather than *exercise*. The term *physical activity* encompasses fitness, exercise, training, and conditioning. The important take-home point is that you need to move. Move in any manner you can tolerate. Anything you do to increase your energy expenditure will help cure your pain and also help with weight loss that will help lessen the stress on your back. All my other chapters have included detailed discussions about aerobic exercise and resistance training. If you are interested, then you can refer to those sections. But your goals are different. Your physical limitations are different. So this chapter is different.

Warm-up for 10 minutes before starting each exercise session.

Aerobic exercise for 10 minutes 3 days a week initially as tolerated. Your goal is to walk for 30 minutes 3–4 days a week.

Resistance (weight) training as directed by your physical therapist. Start with the core-strengthening exercises included in this book. Once you master the easy one, progress to the more difficult.

Cooldown for 10 minutes.

WARM-UP

The warm-up period is one of the most important parts of your activity program because it helps your body prepare for the rigors of exercise and prevents injury.

Start with an easy walk and progress to a brisk pace with your arms swinging. This will gradually increase your body temperature and literally warm up your muscles and your joints. You want to get your blood flowing and your heart pumping. As you warm up your body, you will warm up your muscles, tendons, and ligaments, which will help prevent injury. I think the best warm-up is simply walking outside in the fresh air at a progressively faster pace.

If you have any problem or painful areas, then this is a good time to give them a bit of tender loving care—make sure you do specific stretches for these trouble areas. Your physical therapist will provide these exercises for you.

AEROBIC EXERCISE

Start small. The most important step you will take is your first one. Walking even 10 minutes a day can lead to significant improvement in your aerobic conditioning and pain reduction. If your pain is aggravated by activity, then it becomes easy to avoid movement if you anticipate that it will cause you pain. Avoidance can be appropriate in the short term for acute pain (but only for 1–2 days), but it is not appropriate for chronic pain when your pain is no longer a signal of injury.

You have significantly reduced your activity because of your pain (often subtle, often unaware). So your most important goal is to maintain or return to your normal activity level. Your goal is to reverse the deconditioning that has occurred. You will be surprised how you have subtly avoided movements that hurt. Favoring your pain results in profound muscle and postural imbalances, which only make your pain worse over the years. So ask your spouse or friends to watch you during the day. They will tell you when you're guarding your painful neck or back. Each time you limit your range of motion to prevent discomfort, you are shortening your muscles, weakening them, and causing them to go into spasm. Now not only do you have arthritis in your neck or back causing pain, you have added muscle weakness and spasm, which can easily double the pain you experience. You didn't do it on purpose, but we know that up to 80% of chronic pain has resulted from this vicious cycle of inactivity. As your pain worsens, you move less and the cycle continues. And it will continue until you start to slowly fight your pain and regain your strength and mobility.

Use pain as your guide for how long you should walk. But remember mild pain is not a sign that your are pushing too hard, and it does not signal damage. In chronic pain, your pain signals have taken on a life of their own and don't relate to any damage to muscle, discs, or nerves; they are the expression of your pain disease. If you slowly and carefully increase the duration of your exercise, then you will soon find that you can do much more without any flare of your pain. The best way to get your pain under control is with aerobic exercise. Aerobic exercises are all the exercises that end in -ing. They include *walking, biking, dancing,* and *stair climbing.* The only -ing words that don't count are *sitting* and *lying down.* They won't do a darn thing for your heart or for your pain except make it worse. The only way this program will work for you and your life is to find something that you enjoy.

Often chronic pain patients do best simply by increasing their daily activity level. By fighting muscle wasting and disuse, you will often see rapid results from simple increases in walking or household chores. There is no data that shows that one type of exercise is superior to another to treat pain or prevent its occurrence. It appears that the best advice for chronic pain patients is to just get moving.

If you have severe pain, then you should strongly consider physical therapy as your first step in starting your exercise program. Let the experts teach you safe ways to exercise so that you don't aggravate your problem. But insist that they teach you core-strengthening exercises—stretching is not enough. In fact, stretching alone offers little benefit. If you don't build a strong core to support your back, then it will hurt forever. If you don't get out and walk or swim or bike to improve blood flow to those damaged areas, then they will not get the oxygen they need to heal. It is oxygen that is our life force. If you are in pain and spend your days sitting or lying down afraid to move, then oxygen will never get to the areas that need it the most. Get moving and get the blood flowing. And don't forget the damage your sedentary lifestyle is doing to your heart, lungs, and all your vital organs. You must move it or you will lose it.

I discuss the need to exercise with a strong core in every chapter of this book. But for chronic pain patients, there is nothing more important. As I sit here writing this book, my core is engaged—stomach strong, back tall. It is how you should be sitting while you're reading it; it is how you should sit anytime. And the same holds true for exercise. During your walk, stand tall with your stomach muscles firm to support your back. Try to keep your stomach muscles contracted the entire walk. Think of how you would tense your stomach if someone was going to punch you in the gut. When they come at you with that fist, you don't pull away but instead tighten your stomach to brace for the hit. Or you can try saying *sshhh*. This is another way to tighten your gut and engage the deep core muscles to protect your back. Say it right now loud, and feel your core tighten. The more you *sshhh* yourself, the stronger these critical muscles become and the better you look. Playtex did us no favors by popularizing the girdle. To get the most out of your exercise session, you must be your own Playtex girdle. The girdle did nothing but take away our responsibility for a firm, strong core. By walking with a strong abdomen, you will get four things from each exercise session: pain control, cardiac conditioning, fat burning, and core strengthening. That's a lot of bang for your buck.

You should start your exercise program at a comfortable intensity with minimal pain and slowly increase your intensity over the next six months. It is easy to demand immediate results of yourself and push too hard too fast. But you must provide time for your muscles and joints to adapt. Go slow, go steady, and you will see the results you seek. A very wise man once said, "Infinite patience will yield immediate results." Your results will come, and the benefits will be beyond your wildest dreams, benefits that arise from your willingness to take control of your life and your health and, most importantly, from your belief that you are worth the effort.

Exercise helps treat pain on many other levels as well. Pain is often associated with stress, anxiety, and sleeplessness. Exercise is an effective treatment for all three problems. You can combat not only the physical side of pain, but also the psychological upset that is associated with chronic pain.

Exercise by itself is crucial for treatment of chronic pain. Exercise with weight loss to achieve your desired weight is ideal. Think of the strain that extra 30 lb. around your middle is placing on your poor aching back. My exercise program for my chronic pain patients focuses on activity and weight loss. It has to for success. So put the muffin away, do a few deep knee bends in front of the refrigerator instead, and let's take the first steps.

RESISTANCE EXERCISES

I send all my pain patients for physical therapy after I have controlled their pain. Physical therapists are the safest and most effective way for you to learn appropriate exercises to do at home. Remember, you want to learn strengthening exercises, not just stretches. How much benefit you receive from physical therapy is dependent on the quality of your therapist.

I have only included my favorite core exercises instead of a full resistance program because your therapist should be directing that part of your exercise. You want their close supervision to ensure your success. But after reading this chapter, you now understand what the goals of your therapy session should be. Not an hour spent with what I call lovey-dovey rubbing by the therapist but an hour watching how you move and teaching you how to get stronger and pain-free safer.

The goal of the following exercise program is aimed at improving trunk mobility, trunk and leg strength, force, and endurance. Long-term adherence to an active lifestyle is an acknowledged problem in the general population and is no different in individuals with chronic pain. But your body is screaming for you to take better care of it. Isn't it time you listen?

CORE

Although you'll see everyone in the gym dropping to do 50 sit-ups, they are defeating the purpose on several fronts. The first problem is the number 50. Any exercise you do where you can do more than 20 is not building strength efficiently. Your best bet is to slow down the exercise so you recruit more muscle fibers and build strength efficiently. Doing 50 sit-ups does not provide enough muscle resistance to build strength. Working your abs slowly or adding weight will recruit the maximal number of muscle fibers and provide optimal strength gains. Find 1 or 2 exercises that are hard enough that you can only do 15–20 reps. Even more important for patients with low back pain is the strain 50 crunches puts on your spine. With each abdominal crunch, you compress the discs between your vertebrae. That's a risk for further injury.

The second problem is with the word *sit-up*. It's a bad choice of an exercise to build core strength. You see, any exercise where you raise your body up from the floor is using your hip flexor muscles far more than it uses your abdominal muscles. So with the classic sit-up, you are training your hip flexors but not your abdominal/core muscles. The exercises that follow are safe for your back and will develop all four of your abdominal muscles, providing the strong core you need. Your core muscles include your rectus abdominis muscle, which is your six-pack. But there are three other sets of muscles that run underneath the rectus muscles. These three sets of muscles run diagonally and across your belly and are the ones we want to strengthen. Core also includes your low back muscles. They work in tandem with your abdominal muscles to provide support for your back. Pick a combination of exercises from the list below that work both.

You should start with 2-3 exercises from the list below. As your pain subsides, you can add more for an aggressive core-strengthening program. After 4–6 weeks, switch exercises.

...on your belly, chin on the floor, arms stretched back alongside your body with palms down. With your toes pointed, lift your right leg a few inches off the floor. Hold for several seconds, then slowly lower. Do 3–6 reps; switch legs and repeat (targets back).

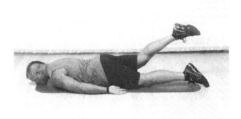

Pelvic Tilt

On the floor, lie on your back with your knees bent. Your feet are flat on the floor and your arms at your sides, palms facing the ground. To a count of 2, slowly roll your pelvis so that hips and lower back are off the floor while upper back and shoulders remain in place. Hold for a count of 2, then slowly lower. Repeat 10 times, or as tolerated (targets back, glutes, and abs).

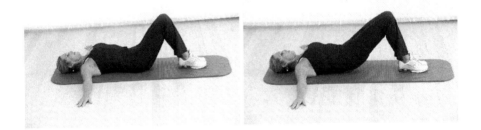

Seated Balance

Sit with knees bent and feet on the floor. Extend your arms in front of you at shoulder level. Engage your abdominal muscles (punched in the gut), and lean back from the hips, keeping your back straight and your chest lifted. Lift your left leg off the floor without moving your pelvis.

Return the starting position and repeat with your left leg. For added difficulty, lift both legs at once. Do a total of 12–15 reps with each leg (targets abdominals, lower back).

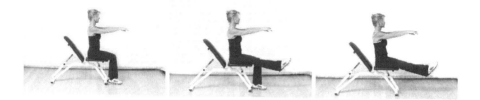

Medicine Ball Twist

Sit on the floor with your legs extended and your back straight. Place a medicine ball (start with a light ball) next to your right hip. Twist and pick up the ball and place it beside the opposite hip. Repeat on each side for a total of 12–15 reps.

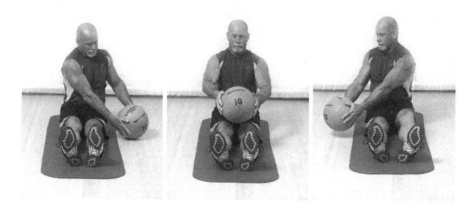

Suitcase Walk

Hold a 3 or 5 lb. dumbbell in your right hand at your side. Keeping your body in perfect alignment, walk as far as you can without discomfort. Repeat with the dumbbell in the other hand. Walk progressively longer distances to challenge your core. Stand tall with stomach strong and shoulders back. Remember to check yourself by saying *sshhh*. This will engage your core the correct way. Increase the amount of weight you carry as the exercise gets easier (targets core-stabilizing muscles).

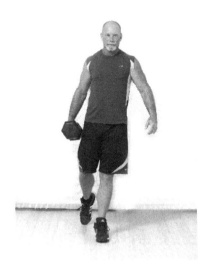

Resistance One-Leg Crunch

Lie on your back with your knees bent with your feet on the floor. Lift your right knee and resist the movement with your right arm. Hold for a count of 2 and then return to the starting position. Repeat on the left. That is 1 repetition. Work up so you can do 8–12 reps (targets abs).

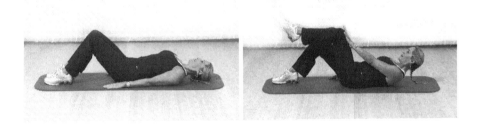

Crunch with Straight Leg

Lie on your back with your knees bent and your arms up over your head. Extend your right leg on the floor. Curl up and bring both arms from overhead to meet your extended leg. Pause for the count of 2 and return to the starting position. Do 8–12 reps on the right and then repeat with the left leg (targets abs).

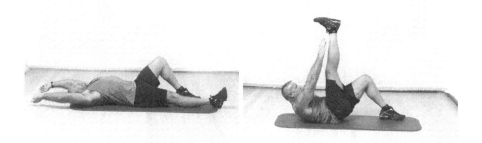

My Crunch

Lie on the floor; with fingers lightly behind your ears, slowly raise your shoulders and buttocks at the same time. If you are doing the exercise correctly, then you will feel your lower abdominal muscles along with your six-pack engage. It is more important to try to lift your buttocks off the floor than lift your shoulders. Hold for 2 seconds and slowly return to your starting position (targets abs).

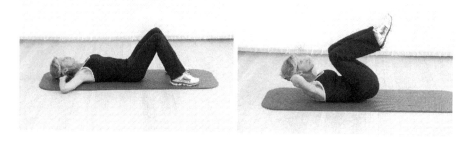

The Bridge

Lie on your back with your knees bent and feet by your buttocks. Stretch your arms down by your sides for balance. Slowly raise your hips as far as you can while keeping your upper back on the floor. Try to form a straight line from your knees to your shoulders. Hold for 3–5 seconds and slowly lower to the floor. Do 12–15 times (targets abdominals, back, hamstrings, and glutes).

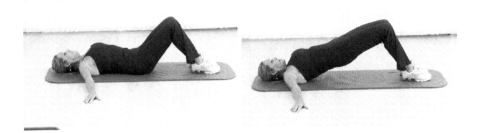

Superman

This works your back extensor muscles with minimal stress on your spine compared to more traditional back exercises.

Kneel on your hands and knees. Keep your stomach tight (like you're being punched), but keep the normal arch in your lower back. Straighten your right leg behind you, keeping it at hip level. Then raise your right arm so it extends straight out at ear level. Keep both your outstretched arm and leg parallel to the floor. Hold for a count of 4, then repeat on the other side. Do 6–8 repetitions each side (targets lower back, glutes, and hamstrings).

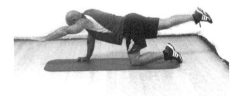

When that becomes simple, start from a standard push-up position and raise your left leg while maintaining the perfect push-up position. Repeat with the right leg. Work up to a total of 8–10 reps per side (targets abdominals, back, hamstrings, and glutes).

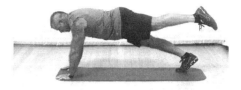

Plank

This is one of my favorite core-strengthening exercises.

Assume a modified push-up position with your forearms resting on the floor. Elbows should be under your shoulders and bent at 90 degrees. Keep your torso steady and your body in a straight line from your head to your toes. Do not let your stomach sag. Hold for as long as you can. Your goal is to hold this for 30 seconds (targets core-stabilizing muscles).

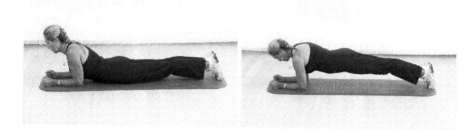

Dryland Swimming

Lie on your stomach on an exercise pad (you might want a towel under your hips for comfort) with your arms extended overhead. Lift your arms and legs off the floor at the same time so they are about 6–8 inches off the ground. Keep looking at the floor. Kick your legs up and down like you are swimming. While you are kicking, move your arms from above your head to your sides and back over your head. Kick for as long as you can, avoiding soreness in your low back (targets back, glutes, and legs).

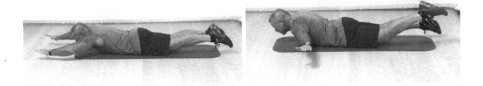

Medicine Ball Trunk Rotation

Lie on your back with your knees bent at a 90-degree angle and your feet in the air. Extend your arms out at shoulder level on the floor. Keep your shoulders flat on the floor and your arms straight out to the sides with your palms down. Rotate your lower body till your bottom leg touches the floor. Hold for 5 seconds and feel the stretch. Then rotate your legs back to center. Keep your legs in the same position throughout the exercise.

When this becomes easy, add a light medicine ball (3 or 5 lb.) and hold it between your legs during the entire exercise. Don't let it drop (targets abs).

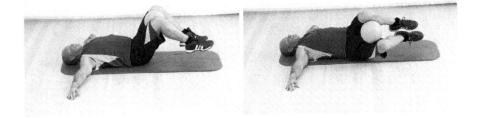

Bicycle

Lie on your back and lift your legs straight in the air. Keep your hands on your stomach to make sure it stays strong and your back stays flat on the floor. Move your legs like you are pedaling a bike. Do this for 30 seconds (targets abs).

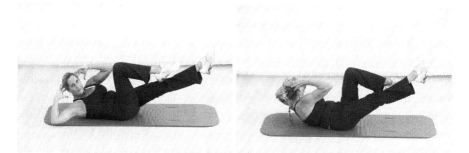

BALANCE

Balance work is especially important for chronic pain patients. Select 2–3 exercises and select new ones every 4–6 weeks.

Marching in Place

Stand tall with your core strong (say *sshhh* to engage your abdominal muscles). March in place slowly, lifting your knees as high as you can. When this is easy, do it on a folded towel or soft cushion.

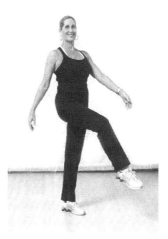

Eyes Closed

Stand on a thick folded towel with your feet shoulder width apart. Stand tall with your abdominal muscles engaged (say *sshhh* to engage them). Close your eyes and visualize the upright position.

Balance on One Leg

Stand with your hand on a chair or bar for support. Shift your weight to your left leg and lift the right leg off the floor. Try letting go of your support or only resting your fingertips on the bar for balance. Your goal is to stand on one leg for 30 seconds. Turn around and repeat it standing on your right leg.

Advanced

Fold a bath towel several times over, place it on the floor, and stand on the center of the towel. This will give you a slightly unstable surface because the towel is soft.

Advanced

Try doing the one-leg balance with your eyes shut. Keep the chair back close so you can steady yourself as needed.

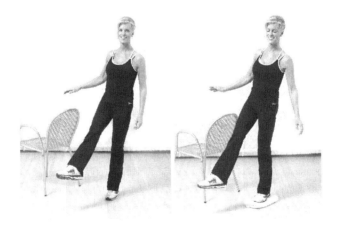

Toe-Stand Balance

Stand facing a sturdy chair or bar with your hands resting lightly on it. Rise up onto your toes and try to let go of the chair and balance for a count of 10. When you are an expert on 2 legs, raise up on our toes and shift your weight to the right leg. Try to balance on your toes on one leg. You will feel the muscles of your entire leg and your core engage. Keep your head high and stomach strong (say *sshhh*).

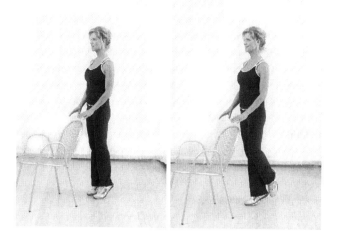

Advanced One-Leg Balance

Stand next to a chair or bar with your right arm resting on it. Slowly lift your left leg behind you. Let your body tilt forward so that you maintain a straight line from the tip of your head to your toes. This will mean that you have to engage your back and stomach muscles to hold your position firm. Bend forward till you are at a 45-degree angle and balance there for 10 seconds. Then if you have the flexibility, continue to tip your body forward until you are looking at the ground and your left leg is extended straight behind you. Balance there for 10 seconds, then slowly return to a stand. Repeat on the right. Work up so you can do 10 on each side without holding on for balance.

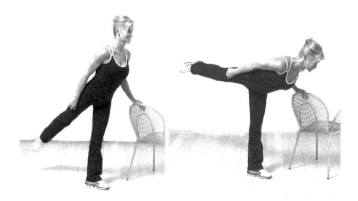

COOLDOWN

The cooldown is important to minimize muscle soreness and fatigue. During exercise, your body accumulates lactic acid (a by-product of muscle work). We associate lactic acid buildup with muscle soreness. The cooldown period gives your body a chance to clear the lactic acid from your muscles and so minimizes postworkout discomfort. With chronic pain, you have more than your share of muscle soreness; I don't want your exercise session to add to it.

Do not stop exercising abruptly. If you simply stop after exercising vigorously, then there is a good chance your blood pressure will drop and you will get light-headed and dizzy. Keep moving. It's what all the experts say and for very good reason. Think of the cooldown period as "active rest" where you are gently returning your body to its pre-exercise state.

Walk slowly for about 5–10 minutes after you finish exercising to gently return your heart rate to its resting level. Or you can simply do a slower version of whatever exercise you were doing. Continue walking until you are breathing normally and can easily carry on a conversation. During your cooldown period is the best time to stretch. But wait until your heart rate has slowed and is approaching your resting rate.

GENERAL STRETCHES FOR YOUR COOLDOWN

Maintaining flexibility of your muscles will increase your range of motion and provide agility. It is also important to minimize injury. When you do the static stretches, start slowly, breathe deeply, and push just to the limit of pain. You will find that as your joint warms up, you will be able to go a little farther each time. Use your breath to help you relax into each stretch. Take a slow, deep breath in through your nose and then relax into the stretch as you exhale through your mouth. Think about your breath and consciously breathe deep in through your nose, filling your lungs down to their bases. This will help you relax and make the most of each stretch. Bouncing or forcing the stretch is actually counterproductive. *Do not bounce.* Plan to do the majority of your stretching program while you are cooling down, while your muscles are still warm from exercising.

Low back pain can result or be aggravated by muscle imbalance in your back and legs. That is where stretching becomes therapeutic. It will help correct these imbalances. This is a very simple start. Your physical therapist will gladly direct you.

Kneeling Quad Stretch

Kneel with your right leg bent in front of you with your knee at a 90-degree angle and your left knee on a mat for cushioning. Keep your body vertical and gently press your hips forward to feel a stretch in the front of the left thigh and hip. Hold for a count of 10, then relax. Repeat 5–10 times and then repeat on the other side.

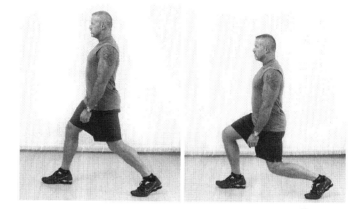

Quadriceps Standing Stretch

Stand facing a chair, holding on to the back lightly for balance. Bend the right knee and grab your ankle with your right hand. Hold for a count of 5, exhaling during the stretch. Try to balance by lifting your hands off the back of the chair on during the stretch to engage core strengthening.

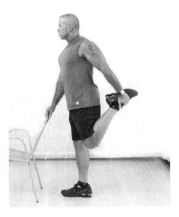

Piriformis Stretch

Lying on your back, bend your right knee with your knee at a 90-degree angle and your foot on the floor. Rest your left ankle on your right leg and let your knee relax out to the side. Gently pull your right knee to your chest and feel the stretch in the left buttock. Hold for a count of 5, exhaling during the stretch.

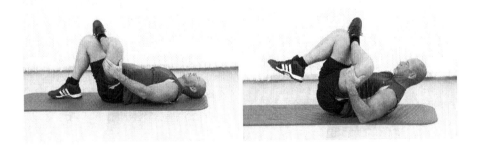

Lying Hamstring Stretch

Lie on your back with both legs straight on the floor and arms by your sides. Bring your right knee to your chest. Place both hands behind your right knee and slowly straighten your right leg. It is OK if you need to lower your right leg to get your knee straight. Hold the straight-leg position for a count of 5, slowly exhaling while you straighten it. Bend the knee again and repeat the exercise 5–10 times on each side.

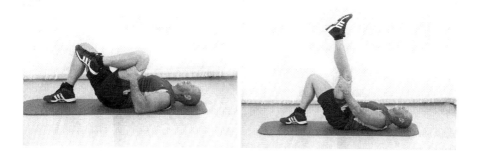

Calf Stretch

Stand on a bottom stair, holding on to the railing for support. Edge your feet back so your heels are off the step. Slowly rise up on your toes and hold for a count of 2. Then lower your body, keeping your knees straight until your heels are below the step and you feel a stretch up the back of your leg.

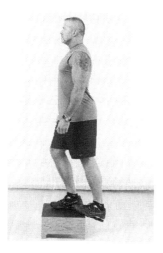

The Cat

Kneel on all fours. Slowly round your back, tucking your head and bringing your shoulders as close as you can to your hips. Pause for the count of 2 and return to the starting position. Then slowly arch your back. Pause and return to the neutral starting position. That is 1 repetition. Do 10 repetitions.

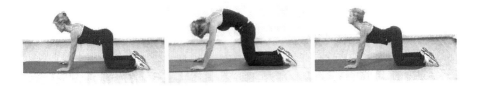

Trunk Twister

Lie on your back on the floor with your arms extended out at shoulder level. Raise your right leg until your toes point to the ceiling. Keeping your leg straight and your shoulders glued to the floor, slowly lower your leg across your body until your toe touches the floor on the left side of your body. Pause at the point that your shoulder wants to lift off the floor. Raise your leg back up in the air and then lower it to the floor. Repeat with your left leg. Do 5–10 repetitions on each side.

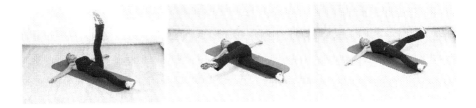

Hamstrings

Lie on your back with your arms out to the side. Raise your right leg into the air. Keeping your knee straight, point and flex your foot 8 times. This will provide a nice stretch for your hamstrings while keeping your back safe. Repeat on the left.

For an extra stretch, grab on to the back of your thigh and gently pull your leg toward you. Breathe in and hold for a count of 2 as you exhale.

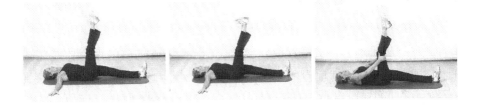

Floor Chest Stretch

Lie faceup on a foam roll with your head supported. Extend your arms out to your sides with your palms facing the ceiling. You will feel a stretch across your chest. Take slow, easy breaths and hold the stretch for 30 seconds. Repeat 3 times.

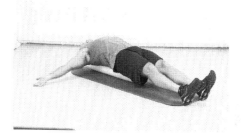

Supine Tuck and Curl

Lie flat on your back, knees bent and feet on the floor. Moving slowly, tilt your pelvis and lift your hips off the floor slightly, then lower. Do 6 reps.

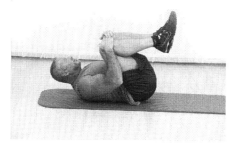

Knee-to-Chest Pose

Lie on your back with your legs fully extended. Draw one knee to your chest and hold it with both hands. Breathe in, and as you breathe out, pull your knee to your chest. Hold for 3–5 breaths. Switch legs and repeat.

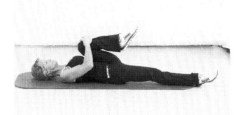

I believe the wise men who say that we are masters of our own fate. Our life is ours, our health is ours, our happiness is ours. Once you take responsibility for your health, you have the power to change it. Stop blaming, stop complaining, and slowly, with love and tenderness, pick yourself up off the couch and go for your first walk. It is the walk of your lifetime.

Exercise to Treat Osteoporosis

The only things known to prevent osteoporosis are a healthy diet and regular exercise. How's that for being master of your own fate? Once again, you have the power to change how you live and how you grow old.

Osteoporosis is defined as a bone mineral density below normal (2.5 standard deviations below the normal level of young adults). Osteoporosis is called brittle bone disease because that is exactly what has happened. Over time your bones become brittle and break easily because there is an imbalance between how much bone is made and how much bone is broken down. This low bone mineral density means that it is very easy to break a bone with a simple fall or twist the wrong way.

Osteoporosis is the most common disease of the skeleton and affects between 7–10 million women and another 2 million men. It's safe to say that we are all potentially at risk. If you are a 50-year-old woman, then your chance of suffering an osteoporotic fracture in your lifetime (usually your spine or your hip) is already 54%, and it only gets higher the older you get. In people who have osteoporosis, hip fractures usually occur because of a fall. Spine fractures, called compression fractures, occur when your vertebrae are compressed, and these can happen as easily as a sneeze. I have a patient who simply looked up to watch a bird fly overhead and suffered a compression fracture of her thoracic spine.

Over 1.3 million fractures occur each year because of osteoporosis. Don't make the same poor choices our mothers and grandmothers have made. An inactive life leads to brittle bones. Let's get on track and strengthen them. It's never too late to start exercising. And even if you have waited till after menopause when this bone loss accelerates at a deadly pace, you can still strengthen your bones with exercise. A diet high in calcium, vitamin D, and regular exercise all help to shift the balance toward bone building and bone strength. Combine these interventions with current medications to promote bone growth, and you can do nothing but win. I hope you are one of the lucky that is ready to take action to avoid this terrible scenario. I hope you are ready to start exercising to fight your disease.

WHY EXERCISE?

You might mistakenly think that exercise could cause your brittle bones to break. But just the opposite is true. Aerobic exercise and muscle strengthening do just the opposite—they build strong bones. So after you have been diagnosed with osteoporosis or osteopenia (borderline brittle), you must start exercising, and you can do it safely. Just follow my direction. Your doctor knows that strengthening effects of exercise on your bones is far greater than the actual change in your BMD score as measured by your bone scan. In fact, a small increase in your BMD is associated with an increase in bone strength of 64%–87%. That's a lot of strengthening. On the flip side, we also know that inactivity is a major risk factor for hip fractures. Elderly men and women who are inactive are more than twice as likely to sustain a hip fracture as those who are physically active. Move it or lose it, like I always say.

Exercise can prevent bone loss, and it can also play a major role in reversing the loss once it's started. With this disease, it is never too late to make an impact. So what can you change? First, get a bone density scan if you haven't already. You will find out if you are normal (safe so far), osteopenic (already sliding down the slippery slope), or osteoporotic (you've already slid). Even if you are osteoporotic, there are many medications now available that can make a significant difference as will exercise and diet. This is one area where modern medicine can actually treat your disease. Please involve your physician in case you need hormone replacement therapy or bisphosphonates to treat your low BMD. Bisphosphonates may be effective in preventing osteoporotic fractures, and we suspect that estrogen may help your bones respond favorably to the mechanical stress of exercise. Talk to your doctor.

DIET CONSIDERATIONS

Dietary factors that can impact your bone density include adequate calcium and vitamin D and the avoidance of excessive caffeine and alcohol consumption. You have to take in enough calcium so that your bones have the building blocks they need to get big and strong. It's just like eating protein when you want to build muscle mass. A dose of 1,000–1,200 mg calcium a day is recommended to minimize postmenopausal bone loss. And vitamin D is necessary for that calcium absorption to occur. You can get sufficient vitamin D with 15 minutes of sun exposure a day (15 minutes without sunscreen is safe). But if you're not getting it, then you need a calcium supplement that contains vitamin D. Caffeine is the bad boy because it increases the amount of calcium lost in your urine, and because of this, it is associated with an increased risk of fracture in elderly women. Alcoholism is also associated with increased urinary loss of calcium and is a risk factor for osteoporosis. Lastly, both low body weight and smoking are also associated with low bone density.

BEFORE YOU BEGIN

Before starting any exercise program, you should get clearance from your doctor. Sounds familiar, I know. But it is much more than a way for me to cover my legal behind. Patients with osteoporosis often have underlying heart disease and hypertension. And, although there are risks when patients with high blood pressure and heart disease exercise, the risks of *not* exercising far outweigh the risks of activity. So you don't get to use your other medical problems as an excuse for not starting. I discuss how to get started safely and the things to watch out for while you are exercising in the chapters devoted to these diseases. If you are a man over the age of 45 or a woman over the age of 50, then it is strongly recommended that you have a stress test before starting an exercise program. These recommendations are from the American College of Sports Medicine based on the prevalence of heart disease in this country. Please check with your doctor. These recommendations are for first-time exercisers. While you're waiting for that doctor's appointment, I encourage you to start your walking program. Light activity is the perfect way to start and is not associated with increased cardiac risk. In fact, that is how I will tell you to start your program anyway.

SAFETY PRECAUTIONS FOR PATIENTS WITH OSTEOPOROSIS

Exercise is one of the best things to stimulate bone growth. But not all exercise is safe when you have osteoporosis. Exercise recommendations for osteoporosis depend on how brittle your bones are. If your bone mineral density is normal, then you should start an aggressive preventative program. If you are on the low end of normal, what we call osteopenic, then you can safely exercise using my direction, but you need to use caution and a few smarts. However, if you have been diagnosed with osteoporosis and/or have suffered an osteoporotic bone fracture, then you should put this book down and start your exercise under the supervision of a physical therapist. At this late stage of the disease, it is not safe for you to exercise without in-depth instruction on balance and safe exercise technique.

Here are important exercise precautions for persons with osteoporosis and osteopenia:

1. There are certain exercises that you should avoid. These are activities that put high-stress loads onto the skeleton such as jumping, running, or jogging. They are contraindicated in people with osteoporosis because of the high compressive forces they impart to the spine and lower extremities. If you have been told you are osteopenic (on your way to becoming osteoporotic), then you should discuss with your doctor whether high-impact activities like running or jogging would be safe for you. Because they deliver high forces to the skeleton, they are very good at stimulating bone growth, but those high forces can be dangerous for those who already have brittle bones. Your doctor will know.

2. You should avoid exercises that require forward bending or twisting at the waist. Bending and twisting produce very high compressive forces over the vertebrae and can cause fractures. So you should avoid toe touches, sit-ups, or rowing exercises. You should also avoid activities that cause these movements such as bowling, golf, and tennis. And my recommendation for my osteoporotic patients is to only do weight lifting exercises under the direct supervision of a physical therapist so you have a trained eye monitoring your form.

3. Lastly, avoid any activities that could increase your chance of falling. Stay off your kid's trampoline; avoid step aerobics and skating (ice and in-line), please. Mall walking provides a safe environment with a smooth surface, so you don't have to worry about tripping on uneven pavement outside.

But what about the milder stages of the disease? That is the focus of the exercise portion of this chapter. If you have been diagnosed with osteopenia or just want a hedge against the normal decline in bone mass that happens with age, then you can make a significant impact on your health with your own exercise program. So let's get moving. The rest of the chapter outlines an efficient and effective program to fight this disease.

LET'S GET STARTED: YOUR EXERCISE PROGRAM

As we've discussed, a well-rounded exercise program includes four components: aerobic exercise, strength training, balance, and flexibility. The impact of walking, dancing, and hiking all stimulate bone growth. And just as important is the impact of muscles pulling against bones as you lift weights. So aerobic exercise and weight training are equally important if you have osteoporosis. A third consideration is a program to improve your balance. If you don't practice balance, then you will lose it too. Here is the outline of your exercise program:

Warm-up for 10 minutes before starting each exercise session; include stretching exercises.

Aerobic exercise for 10 minutes 3 days a week initially, then progress to 30 minutes 3–4 days a week over the next 2–3 months. Start at an intensity of 4–5 on the Borg scale if you are new to exercise. Work up to an intensity that is 60%–70% of your maximum.

Resistance (weight) training for 20–30 minutes, 3 days a week to supplement your aerobic work. Do 12–15 reps of each exercise using a weight load that stresses your muscles but never sacrifices perfect form. And don't forget the balance exercises.

Cooldown for 10 minutes after each session; don't forget to stretch.

WARM-UP (5-10 minutes before every exercise session)

The warm-up period is one of the most important parts of your exercise program because it helps your body prepare for the rigors of exercise and prevents injury.

Start with an easy walk and progress to a brisk pace with your arms swinging. This will gradually increase your body temperature and literally warm up your muscles and your joints. You want to get your blood flowing and your heart pumping. As you warm up your body, you will warm up your muscles, tendons, and ligaments, which will help prevent injury.

I think the best warm-up is simply walking outside in the fresh air for 10 minutes at a progressively faster pace. By the time the 10 minutes is done, you should be breathing harder and feel that your body is warm. Another way to warm up is to do an exercise-specific warm-up where you do one set of your weight lifting exercises using about half the weight you will train with during your exercise session.

AEROBIC EXERCISE (30-40 minutes 3-4 days a week)

So where do you start? Walk. Everyone should walk. It is a good yet safe impact exercise. You should start your walking program slowly and simply. If you are new to exercise, then start with just 10–15 minutes a day for 2–4 weeks to allow your muscles and joints to adapt. Your goal is to work up to 30 minutes of brisk walking (or other impact aerobic exercise) 3–4 days a week. If fat loss is also a concern, then increase your exercise duration to 40 minutes. Add to these numbers a 10-minute warm-up and 5–10 minute cooldown. If osteopenia is your only medical problem, then you should work up to a moderate exercise intensity of 60%–70% max (breathing heavily but you can still talk) over the next several months. If you have been sedentary and are beginning an exercise program for the first time, then you should start at a very low intensity (40%–50% maximum or a perceived exertion of 4–5) and gradually increase your effort as tolerated.

Choose exercises that you enjoy. You have made an important life choice when you decided to treat your brittle bones with exercise. So find something that you love to do and keep your commitment strong. Safe and effective activities for people with osteoporosis and osteopenia include walking, hiking, dancing, and stair climbing. You should avoid golf and tennis because of the flexion and twisting forces they place on your spine. Swimming is a great exercise, but because it is not a weight-bearing activity, it does not stimulate bone growth. Water aerobics also fails on this front.

If you are young and healthy (or your doctor tells you that you are healthy enough to act like a 20-year-old) and seeking a preventative program, then the very best activities for stimulating bone growth are high-impact activities like jogging and any activity that involves jumping like basketball or volleyball.

You can think of training your bones just like you think of training your muscles. The best way to train both are by using a variety of exercises that stress the bones and muscles different ways; your bones (and muscles) will strengthen most efficiently if you change up your routine every couple weeks and continually try new exercises. Every organ in your body (bone, muscle, heart, and lungs) requires a long-term commitment to exercise that is progressive in nature. So if you stop exercising, then the benefits you have made in bone strength will recede. You see, your body was made to move. It was not designed to be an adornment for your living room couch.

Remember the following:

1. Gains in bone density will only be maintained as long as you continue to exercise. If you don't use it, then you definitely will lose it.

2. Approximately 9 months to 1 year of exercise are required to see a significant improvement in bone density.

And most importantly, go walking with your daughter. Give her the hedge against this terrible disease that we didn't know about when we were growing up. The more bone mass she can build in her youth, the better chance she has of avoiding osteoporosis as she ages.

RESISTANCE EXERCISES (20–30 minutes 2–3 days a week)

Resistance training is an important part of your bone-strengthening program. The force of muscle pulling against bone that occurs every time you lift weights has been shown to be very effective at stimulating bone growth. So you should divide your time almost equally between aerobic work and weight training. The following exercises are designed for the person with normal or low normal bone mass. Please read the specific cautions to ensure your exercise safety. Every 4–6 weeks, pick new exercises to keep your bones and muscles challenged. Select one or two exercises from each group to provide a complete full-body workout. Plan to do 12–15 reps of each exercise for optimal bone and muscle strengthening. Your form during these exercises must be your primary focus. I want you to do each exercise slowly, watching not only where the weight is moving, but you should also be checking the alignment of your back, hips, and shoulders during each movement. When you are working your legs, make sure that your knees are always over your toes to avoid stress on your knees and hips. The pictures below will illustrate that for you. The balance exercise section is especially important for you to help prevent falls, which can be devastating if you have brittle bones. Balance is like any other skill; if you don't practice, then you will lose it.

Remember, if you have been diagnosed with osteoporosis, not just osteopenia, you should start your exercise program under a physical therapist's supervision. They will watch how you exercise and ensure that you have perfect form so that your exercise improves bone strength rather than weaken it.

CORE

Although you'll see everyone in the gym dropping to do 50 sit-ups, they are defeating the purpose on several fronts. The first problem is the number 50. Any exercise you do where you can do more than 20 is not building strength efficiently. Your best bet is to slow down the exercise so you recruit more muscle fibers and build strength efficiently. Doing 50 sit-ups does not provide enough muscle resistance to build strength. Working your abs slowly or adding weight will recruit the maximal number of muscle fibers and provide optimal strength gains. Find 1 or 2 exercises that are hard enough that you can only do 15–20 reps.

The second problem is with the word *sit-up*. It's a bad choice of an exercise to build core strength. You see, any exercise where you raise your body up from the floor is using your hip flexor muscles far more than it uses your abdominal muscles. So with the classic sit-up, you are training your hip flexors but not your abdominal/core muscles. The sit-up is not only ineffective, but it is also potentially dangerous. It can easily strain your low back, a situation we want to avoid. With each sit-up, you compress the discs between your vertebrae. And if you have osteoporosis, you can compress your vertebral bones themselves.

The exercises that follow are safe for your back and your bones and will develop all four of your abdominal muscles, providing the strong core you need. Your core muscles include your rectus abdominis muscle, which is your six-pack. But there are three other sets of muscles that run underneath the rectus muscles. These three sets of muscles run diagonally and across your belly and are the ones we want to strengthen. We'll call them your core-stabilizing muscles. The following exercises focus on strengthening these. Core also includes your low back muscles. They work in tandem with your abdominal muscles to provide support for your back. Pick a combination of exercises that work both.

You should do 2–3 of the following exercises as part of your weight training program. After 4–6 weeks, switch exercises.

Half Locust

Lie on your belly, chin on the floor, arms stretched back alongside your body with palms down. With your toes pointed, lift your right leg a few inches off the floor. Hold for several seconds, then slowly lower. Do 3–6 reps; switch legs and repeat (targets back).

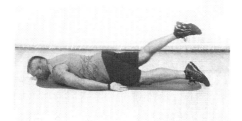

Resistance One-Leg Crunch

Lie on your back with your knees bent with your feet on the floor. Lift your right knee and resist the movement with your right arm. Hold for a count of 2 and then return to the starting position. Repeat on the left. That is 1 repetition. Work up to 8–12 reps with each leg (targets abs).

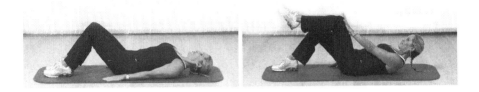

Crunch with Straight Leg

Lie on your back with your knees bent and your arms up over your head. Extend your right leg on the floor. Curl up and bring both arms from overhead to meet your extended leg. Pause for the count of 2 and return to the starting position. Do 8–12 reps on the right and then repeat with the left leg (targets abs).

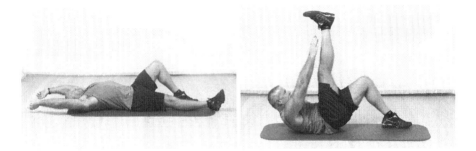

My Crunch

Lie on the floor; with fingers lightly behind your ears, slowly raise your shoulders and buttocks at the same time. If you are doing the exercise correctly, then you will feel your lower abdominal muscles along with your six-pack engage. It is more important to try to lift your buttocks off the floor than lift your shoulders. Hold for 2 seconds and slowly return to your starting position (targets abs).

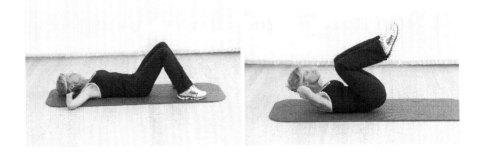

Superman

This works your back extensor muscles with minimal stress on your spine compared to more traditional back exercises.

Kneel on your hands and knees. Keep your stomach tight (like you're being punched), but keep the normal arch in your lower back. Straighten your right leg behind you, keeping it at hip level. Then raise your right arm so it extends straight out at ear level. Keep both your outstretched arm and leg parallel to the floor. Hold for a count of 4, then repeat on the other side. Do 6–8 repetitions each side (targets lower back, glutes, and hamstrings).

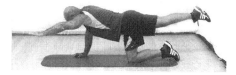

When that becomes simple, start from a standard push-up position and raise your left leg while maintaining the perfect push-up position. Repeat with the right leg (targets abdominals, back, hamstrings, and glutes).

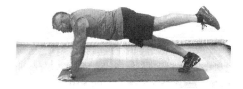

Fitness Ball Crunch

Lie on a fitness ball that is the right size for you. The correct-size ball is one that when you sit on it, your knees are bent at a right angle. Lie back on the ball so your thighs and torso are parallel to the floor. Cross your arms over your chest. In a slow, controlled manner, contract your stomach, lifting your shoulders off the ball, and gently lift your chin toward the ceiling. As you raise your shoulders, slowly exhale. Rise no more than 45 degrees. Then slowly return to your starting position. Inhale as you lower. The closer your feet are together, the harder the exercise.

For beginners, place your shoulders and upper back on the ball with your thighs and torso are parallel to the floor. Do crunches with the stability ball supporting your entire torso. As that gets easy, place the ball farther down your back so that more of your upper body is off the ball. You will find this is a much harder way to do the crunch (targets abs).

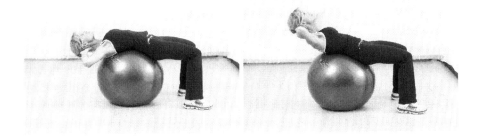

Single-Leg Lowering

Lie on your back with both legs straight up in the air (never lock your knees). Press the small of your back into the floor. It is best to place your hands slightly under the small of your back to make sure it never arches up. Point your foot and slowly lower your right leg as far as you can while maintaining perfect form. Your goal is to lower it 2–3 inches from the floor. Bring your right leg back up and repeat with the left. Do 8–12 reps (targets abs, quads).

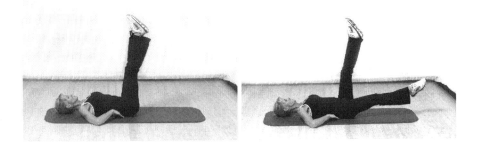

Plank

This is one of my favorite core-strengthening exercises.

Assume a modified push-up position with your forearms resting on the floor. Elbows should be under your shoulders and bent at 90 degrees. Keep your torso steady and your body in a straight line from your head to your toes. Do not let your stomach sag. Hold for as long as you can. Your goal is to hold this for 30 seconds (targets core-stabilizing muscles).

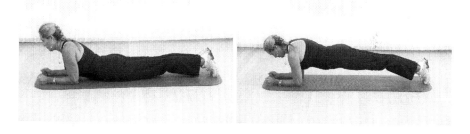

Advanced Plank

Assume a modified push-up position with your forearms resting on the floor. Elbows should be under your shoulders and bent at 90 degrees. Keep your torso steady and your body in a straight line from your head to your toes. Do not let your stomach sag. Raise your right arm and extend it overhead. Keep your body alignment while you hold it out. Return to the starting position. Repeat with the left arm. Work up to 4 repetitions on each side (targets core-stabilizing muscles).

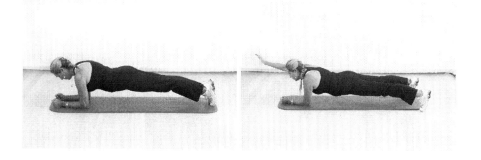

Suitcase Walk

Hold a 3 or 5 lb. dumbbell in your right hand at your side. Keeping your body in perfect alignment, walk as far as you can without discomfort. Repeat with the dumbbell in the other hand. Walk progressively longer distances to challenge your core. Stand tall with stomach strong and shoulders back. Remember to check yourself by saying *sshhh*. This will engage your core the correct way. Increase the amount of weight you carry as the exercise gets easier (targets core-stabilizing muscles).

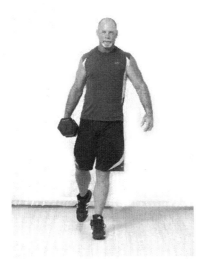

SHOULDERS

Pick 1–2 exercises from this section. Change exercises every 4–6 weeks.

Shoulder Shrug

Stand holding a 3–5 lb. dumbbell in each hand, palms facing toward each other. Shrug your shoulders up to your ears and pause. Slowly lower your shoulders. Repeat 12 times (targets shoulders).

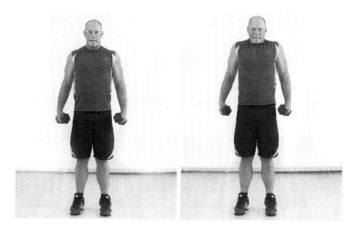

Dumbbell Upright Row

Stand holding a pair of dumbbells in front of your thighs, arms straight and palms facing your body. Lift your upper arms and bring the dumbbells up until your hands are just below your chin. Pause and then lower the weight back to the starting position. Repeat 12 times (targets shoulders).

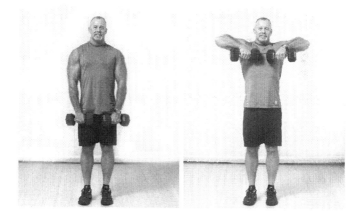

Controlled Fly

Kneel on a bench with your right leg and right arm on the bench. In your left hand you are holding a 1 or 3 lb. weight with the palm facing you. Keep your back flat and stomach strong during the exercise. Slowly lift the weight out to the side till your arm is parallel to the floor. Repeat with the other arm and do 8–12 reps a side (targets shoulders).

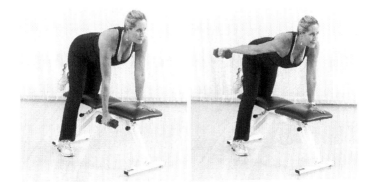

Toss and Catch

Play toss and catch with a beach ball or light medicine ball. As the exercise gets easier, you can increase the weight of the ball. Keep your stomach engaged (tense the muscles like you're going to be punched in the stomach) throughout your game, especially right before you throw the ball (targets shoulders and abs).

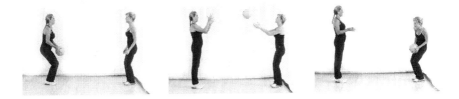

Lateral Raises 3 Ways

This is one of my favorite exercises and part of my exercise routine. To use all three heads of the deltoid, you will do the standard lateral raise using three different hand positions. Do this exercise with low weight and slow, controlled movements.

Stand tall, stomach firm, holding a 1, 3, or 5 lb. dumbbell in each hand. With your hands facing forward and arms straight, slowly raise both dumbbells at a 45-degree angle to shoulder level. Your thumbs should be pointing at the ceiling. Do not raise them above shoulder level. Slowly lower to the count of 2 or 4. You will feel this primarily in the anterior head of the deltoid (your shoulder muscle).

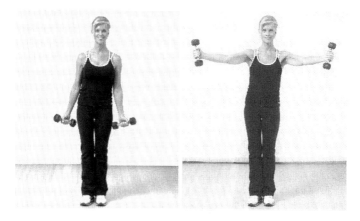

Next, turn your hands to face each other and lift the dumbbells slowly to the side. All your knuckles will be directed toward the ceiling. Do not raise them above shoulder level. This will strengthen the middle head of the deltoid. Slowly lower.

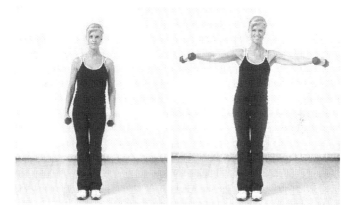

Lastly, turn your hands facing the back with your pinkies on top. Slowly lift to the side, again stopping at shoulder height. You will feel this engage the posterior head of the deltoid. Slowly lower.

Repeat the entire set (all three moves are 1 set) 8 times.

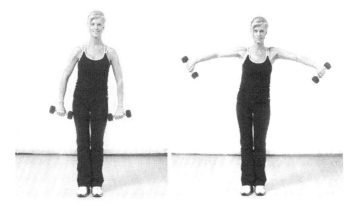

Alternating Shoulder Dumbbell Press

By alternating your arms, you also get core strengthening with the exercise.

Sit with your back supported. Engage your core (like you are preparing to be punched). This will provide a solid core to protect your back and double the value of the exercise by working your stomach muscles. Hold a 1–3 lb. dumbbell in each hand at shoulder level with palms facing each other. Press the dumbbell in your right hand straight above you until your arm is straight and the weight is above your head. Then slowly lower the weight to the starting position. Repeat on the left. Do a total of 8–12 per side (targets shoulders and core).

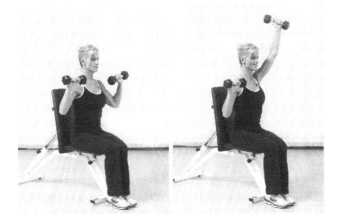

Advanced

Do the same exercise standing or stand on one leg to challenge your core. Keep your abdominal muscles engaged.

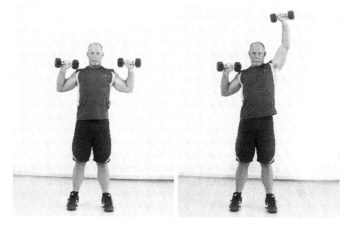

CHEST

Select one exercise from this section and pick new exercises to try every 4–6 weeks.

Wall Push-ups (the perfect beginner's exercise)

Stand at arm's length from the wall. Put both hands on the wall at chest level. Slowly bend your elbows to the count of 4 and then slowly straighten them. Repeat 12 times. When this is easy go to the modified push up below (targets chest).

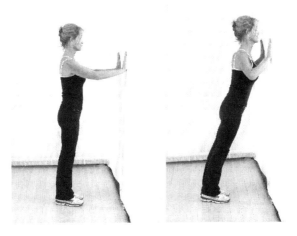

Push-ups on Knees

I know these are girl push-ups, but done correctly, they will result in impressive improvements in your strength. Once you can do 12 of these with perfect form, then it is time to do them in the regular push-up position. Keep your core strong throughout the push-up by maintaining a straight line from your knees to the top of your head.

Kneel on the floor with your knees on a pad. Walk your arms out until your body is in a straight line with your knees bent. In this modified push-up position, I want you to slowly lower your body (keeping a straight line from the tip of your head to your knees) until you are barely touching the floor and then slowly return to the starting position, keeping perfect form (targets chest). Do 6–12 reps in each of the three hand positions illustrated.

A) Normal push-up position—elbows are at a 90-degree angle with your hands right under your elbows.

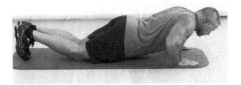

B) Wide-arm position—hands are placed out past your elbows so the angle of your elbows is about 120 degrees.

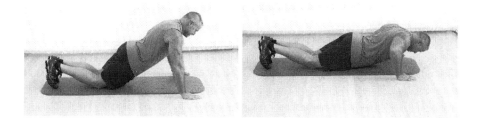

C) Diamond—place your hands so that your thumb and index fingers touch each other and make the shape of a diamond.

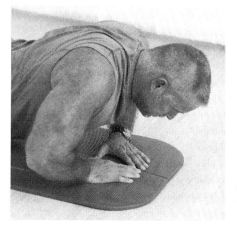

Dumbbell Incline Bench Press

Lie faceup on an incline bench and hold 3-5 lb. dumbbells along the outside of your chest with elbows bent and palms facing inward. Slowly press the weight straight above your chest (see picture). Pause and then slowly lower (targets chest).

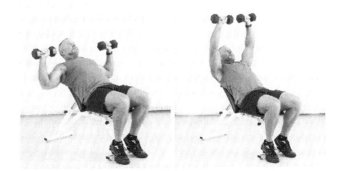

Dumbbell Incline Fly

Lie faceup on an incline bench. Hold 3-5 lb. dumbbells straight over your chest with your palms facing each other. Slowly open your arms, keeping your hands in line with your shoulders. Stop when the weights are level with your chest. Pause and return to the starting position. Repeat 8–12 times (targets chest).

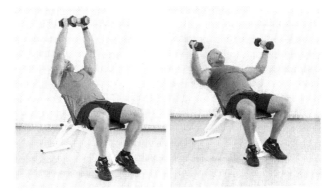

LEGS

Pick one exercise from each of the leg sections: glutes, hamstrings, and calves. The exercises in these sections have good overlap, so you'll be working the same muscles several ways, just with a different focus in each grouping. Start with just one exercise per group and later increase the number to continue to challenge your muscles. Pick a new exercise every 4–6 weeks. And don't forget the balance exercises at the end of this section.

LEGS–QUADS

Sit to Stand

Sit on a firm straight-backed chair. Engage your core (tighten your stomach like someone was going to punch you in the gut). With stomach strong, slowly stand up. Use your legs, not your arms, to lift your body off the chair. If you cannot stand without using your arms, then allow them to assist you—but no more than necessary. Slowly lower back to the seated position, but halfway down, pause for a count of 2 or 4, then continue to the seated position. Do as many as you can with perfect form (targets quadriceps, core).

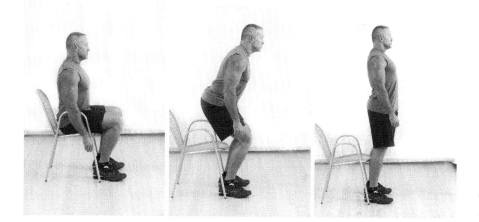

Step Up

Stand straight with your stomach strong. Step your right foot onto first step and slowly straighten leg. Keep toes facing front. Bring left foot up to touch step by right ankle, then slowly lower your weight to count of 4 onto left leg. Don't push off back leg. Move slowly so the muscles, and not the momentum, do the work. As you stand up, press your weight through the heel, not the ball, of your foot. Repeat 10 times on each leg. When the stair step becomes easy, carry 5–10 lb. dumbbells to increase difficulty (targets quadriceps and glutes, balance).

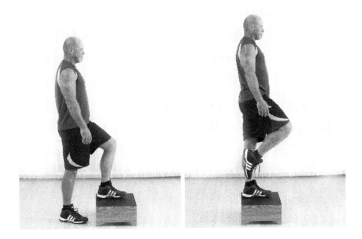

Wall Squat

Stand with a fitness ball between you and a wall. Rest your lower back against the fitness ball. Your feet should be shoulder width apart and about 3 feet away from the wall. Slowly bend your knees till your thighs are parallel to the floor, or as low as you can go. Make sure you keep your knees directly over your toes. Pause and then squeeze your buttocks as you return to the standing position. Build up to 12-15 reps. As this gets easier, deepen your knee bend to optimize quad strengthening. (targets quadriceps, glutes).

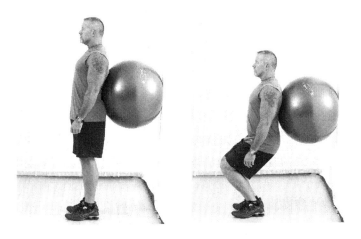

Standing Hip Flexion

Stand next to a chair with your feet together and hold on to the chair with your left hand for support. Bend your right knee and lift it up to your waist, pause, and slowly lower it. Repeat 8-12 times and then turn and do the same thing with the left leg. Then try to do the same exercise without grabbing your leg (targets hip flexors, balance).

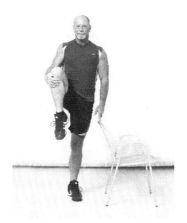

Fitness Ball Single-Leg Squat

Stand facing away from a fitness ball, about 2 feet in front of it. Place your right foot on the ball. With your weight on your left leg, bend your left knee and let your right leg roll back on the ball. Keep your left knee straight over your toes. Pause and return to a stand. Build to 12–15 repetitions with each leg. When this gets easy, hold 3 or 5 lb. dumbbells in your hands (targets quads and glutes, balance).

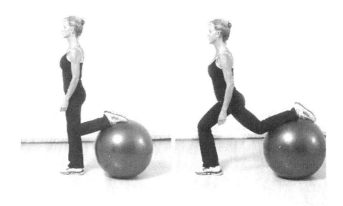

LEGS–HAMSTRINGS

Pick 1–2 exercises from this group. Change exercises every 4–6 weeks.

Hip Bridge

Lying on your back with heels tucked close to your buttocks, lift your buttocks off the ground so your body forms a straight line from knees to shoulders. Hold for 2 seconds, then slowly lower over a 2-second count. Do 8–12 reps (targets hamstrings, glutes, and low back)

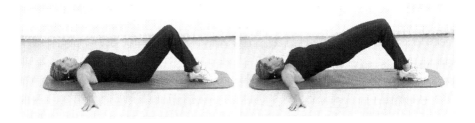

For added difficulty, straighten your right leg from the knee and do the movement using only the left leg to lift your body. Keep the right leg straight during the exercise. Do 8–12 reps on each side.

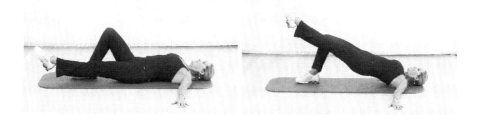

For even more difficulty, straighten your right leg with your toes pointing at the ceiling. Keep your leg pointed toward the ceiling as you raise your body with your left leg. Do 8–12 reps then repeat with the left leg straight.

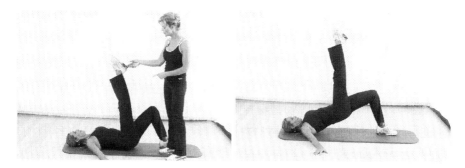

Leg Curl

I prefer this machine because it avoids the potential back stress that can occur when you use the supine leg-curl machine. Sit on the leg-curl machine. Adjust the machine so the lower pad lies behind your ankles and your knees almost straight. Start with a light weight and slowly bend your knees until your ankles are near your buttocks. Pause and then slowly return to the starting position. For added difficulty and to help focus on your hamstrings, try pointing your toes during the movement. Do 8-12 reps (targets hamstrings).

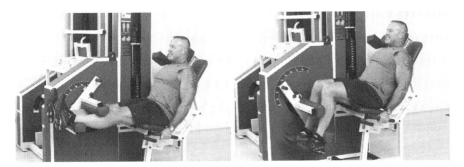

One-Legged Bridge with Crossed Leg

Lie faceup, knees bent, and feet flat on the ground. Cross your right ankle over your left thigh. Let your right knee relax out to the side, but keep hips squared forward. Lift your hips off the ground with your stomach pulled in. Lift hips until you form a straight line from your chest through your hips. Hold for a count of 2 and return to the starting position. Do 12-15 times (targets hamstrings, glutes).

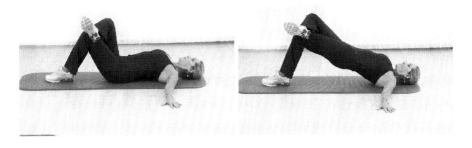

Fire Hydrant

Kneel on all fours on a mat, and place a 1 or 3 lb. weight behind your right knee. Squeeze your leg muscles so that the dumbbell stays locked in place. Keeping your back flat and your head down, slowly raise your right leg until your thigh is parallel with the floor. Pause and then lower your right leg to the starting position. Use a weight that only lets you complete the exercise 10-15 times (targets hamstrings and glutes).

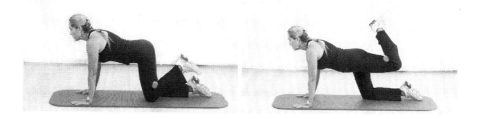

LEGS–CALVES

Pick one of these exercises to start with. Change every 4–6 weeks. And remember that many of the balance exercises strengthen your calves as well.

Seated Calf Raise

Sit with 5 or 10 lb. dumbbells resting on each knee. Slowly lift your knees and come up on the balls of your feet. Pause for a count of 2 and then slowly lower. Make sure that you're using your calves to raise the weights and not your arms. Repeat 12–15 times (targets calves).

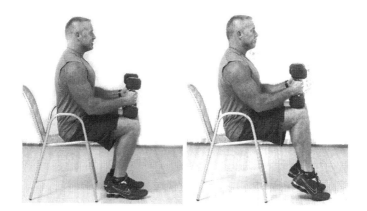

Standing Calf Raise

Stand on a step or a block with the toes and ball of your right foot at the edge of the step. Hold on to a wall or chair with your left hand for balance. Cross your left foot behind your right ankle and balance yourself on the ball of your right foot. Lower your heel as far as you can till you feel a stretch in the back of your calf. Lift your heel as high as you can, pause, and return to the starting position. Do 10–15 reps and repeat with the left leg (targets calves, balance).

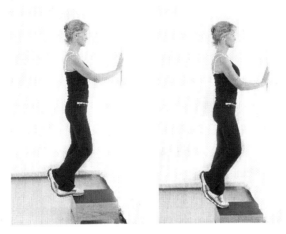

BALANCE

Pick 2–3 exercises from this group. Switch exercises every 4–6 weeks.

Marching in Place

Stand tall with your core strong (say *sshhh* to engage your abdominal muscles). March in place slowly, lifting your knees as high as you can. When this is easy, do it on a folded towel or soft cushion.

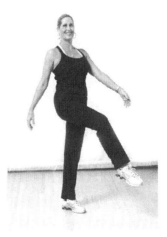

Eyes Closed

Stand on a thick folded towel with your feet shoulder width apart. Stand tall with your abdominal muscles engaged (say *sshhh* to engage them). Close your eyes and visualize the upright position.

Balance on One Leg

Stand with your hand on a chair or bar for support. Shift your weight to your left leg and lift the right leg off the floor. Try letting go of your support or only resting your fingertips on the bar for balance. Your goal is to stand on one leg for 30 seconds. Turn around and repeat it standing on your right leg.

Advanced

Fold a bath towel several times over, place it on the floor, and stand on the center of the towel. This will give you a slightly unstable surface because the towel is soft.

Advanced

Try doing the one-leg balance with your eyes shut. Keep the chair back close so you can steady yourself as needed.

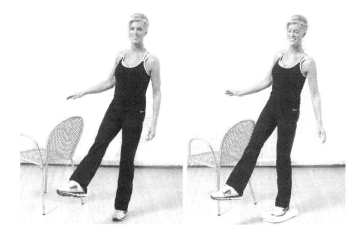

Toe-Stand Balance

Stand facing a sturdy chair or bar with your hands resting lightly on it. Rise up onto your toes and try to let go of the chair and balance for a count of 10. When you are an expert, then raise up on your toes and, still holding on gently, shift your weight to the right leg and try to balance on your toes on one leg. You will feel the muscles of your entire leg and your core engage. Keep your head high and stomach strong (say *sshhh*).

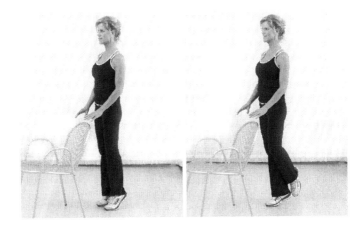

Step-ups on a Stair

Stand straight with stomach strong, holding on to handrail. Step your right foot onto first step and slowly straighten leg. Keep toes facing front. Bring left foot up to touch step by right ankle, then slowly lower your weight to count of 4 onto left leg. Repeat 10 times with each leg. Don't push off back leg. Move slowly so the muscles, and not the momentum, do the work. As you stand up, press your weight through the heel, not the ball, of your foot.

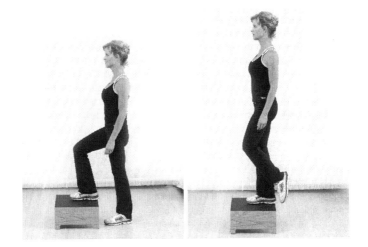

Did you notice that I did not include any specific exercises for your biceps or triceps? I did that on purpose. If you do the exercises I gave you, then they will work your biceps and triceps also. There is no need to waste your time on such small muscle groups. Use your exercise time efficiently and focus on large muscle groups that will improve your strength, burn more calories, and improve your ability to carry out your daily activities. And I promise, your biceps and triceps will look marvelous.

COOLDOWN (5-10 minutes after every exercise session)

Your cooldown is as important as the warm-up phase of your exercise program. Do not stop exercising abruptly. If you simply stop after exercising vigorously, then there is a good chance your blood pressure will drop and you will get light-headed and dizzy. Keep moving. It's what all the experts say and for very good reason. Think of the cooldown period as "active rest," where you are gently returning your body to its pre-exercise state. Walk slowly for about 10 minutes after you finish exercising to gently return your heart rate to its resting level. Or you can simply do a slower version of whatever exercise you were doing. Continue walking until you are breathing normally and can easily carry on a conversation. Your cooldown period is the best time to stretch. But wait until your heart rate has slowed and is approaching your resting value.

GENERAL STRETCHES FOR YOUR COOLDOWN

Maintaining flexibility of your muscles will increase your range of motion and provide agility. It is also important to minimize injury. The most important and permanent way to increase your flexibility is to do every resistance exercise through the full range of movement. Exercises like lunges, squats, and even push-ups should be done by moving your body through its full *pain-free* range of motion. As you move your body as far as it can, make sure you keep good form during every repetition. But because they feel so good, I have included my favorite static stretches. When you do the static stretches, start slowly, breathe deeply, and push just to the limit of pain. You will find that as your joint warms up, you will be able to go a little farther each time. Use your breath to help you relax into each stretch. Take a slow, deep breath in through your nose and then relax into the stretch as you exhale through your mouth. Think about your breath and consciously breathe deep in through your nose, filling your lungs down to their bases. This will help you relax and make the most of each stretch. Bouncing or forcing the stretch is actually counterproductive. *Do not bounce.* Plan to do the majority of your stretching program while you are cooling down, while your muscles are still warm from exercising.

Flexibility is important, but you must be careful to maintain a straight spine (i.e., avoid toe touches). Bending forward or twisting the spine results in large compressive forces and can risk vertebral fracture. I have given you some safe options to start with.

Do these leg exercises to maintain balance between the muscles in the front and back of your hips and legs to minimize low back strain.

Kneeling Quad Stretch

Kneel with your right leg bent in front of you with your knee at a 90-degree angle and your left knee on a mat for cushioning. Keep your body vertical and gently press your hips forward to feel a stretch in the front of the left thigh and hip. Hold for a count of 10, then relax. Repeat 5–10 times and then repeat on the other side.

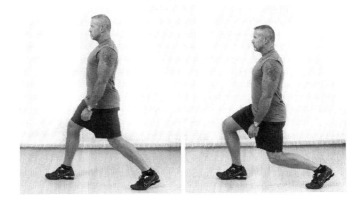

Quadriceps Standing Stretch

Stand facing a chair, holding on to the back lightly for balance. Bend the right knee and grab your ankle with your right hand. Hold for a count of 5, exhaling during the stretch. Try to balance by lifting your hands off the back of the chair on during the stretch to engage core strengthening.

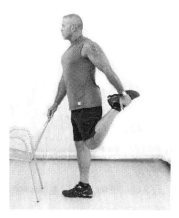

Piriformis Stretch

Lying on your back, bend your right knee with your knee at a 90-degree angle and your foot on the floor. Rest your left ankle on your right leg and let your knee relax out to the side. Gently pull your right knee to your chest and feel the stretch in the left buttock. Hold for a count of 5, exhaling during the stretch.

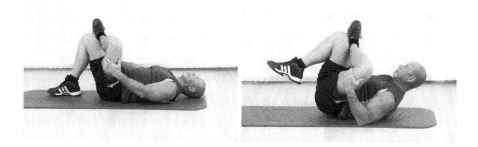

Lying Hamstring Stretch

Lie on your back with both legs straight on the floor and arms by your sides. Bring your right knee to your chest. Place both hands behind your right knee and slowly straighten your right leg. It is OK if you need to lower your right leg to get your knee straight. Hold the straight-leg position for a count of 5, slowly exhaling while you straighten it. Bend the knee again and repeat the exercise 5–10 times on each side.

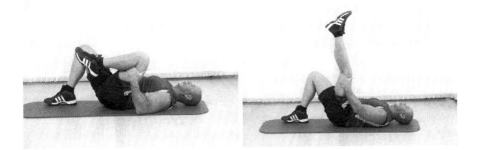

Calf Stretch

Stand on a bottom stair, holding on to the railing for support. Edge your feet back so your heels are off the step. Slowly rise up on your toes and hold for a count of 2. Then lower your body, keeping your knees straight until your heels are below the step and you feel a stretch up the back of your leg.

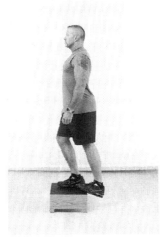

Floor Chest Stretch

Lie faceup on a foam roll with your head supported. Extend your arms out to your sides with your palms facing the ceiling. You will feel a stretch across your chest. Take slow, easy breaths and hold the stretch for 30 seconds. Repeat 3 times.

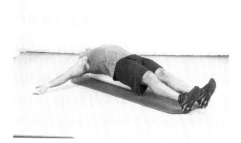

Supine Tuck and Curl

Lie flat on your back, knees bent and feet on the floor. Moving slowly, tilt your pelvis and lift your hips off the floor slightly, then lower. Do 6 reps.

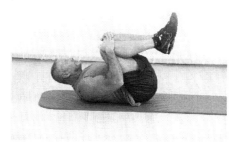

Knee-to-Chest Pose

Lie on your back with your legs fully extended. Draw one knee to your chest and hold it with both hands. Breathe in and, as you breathe out, pull your knee to your chest. Hold for 3–5 breaths. Switch legs and repeat.

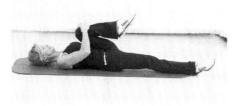

I believe the wise men who say that we are masters of our own fate. Our life is ours, our health is ours, our happiness is ours. Once you take responsibility for your health, you have the power to change it. Stop blaming, stop complaining, and slowly, with love and tenderness, pick yourself up off the couch and go for your first walk. It is the walk of your lifetime.

ABOUT THE AUTHOR

Ruth Anderson, MD, MS, is a noted fitness expert, wellness consultant, and pain management specialist. She combines her extensive medical background with a master's degree in exercise physiology and 25 years of experience in fitness and nutrition, bringing a unique perspective to the world of health. She is board certified in both anesthesiology and pain management. Dr. Anderson (all her patients call her Dr. Ruth) runs her own pain management practice in Palm Desert, California, where she uses her fitness and wellness expertise to teach her patients that the power to heal lies within and provides the tools to help them reach their goals.

This book is an integral part of that teaching. Embodied in this work are all the things she tells each of her patients in a form you can take with you and learn from daily. But the doctor does much more than preach. She has been a chronic pain sufferer since her back injury in 1980 ended her dance career. Dr. Anderson has suffered the frustration of modern medicine's failed attempts to cure her. She knows—there are no cures. But she has learned that diet and exercise can control her pain, and she is now stronger and in less pain than she has been since age 20. She lives the life she preaches. Dr. Ruth has refused to let her pain disease rule her life and will teach you how your hypertension, diabetes, or arthritis doesn't have to rule your lives either.

Made in the USA
Lexington, KY
15 August 2010